LIVING THERAPY SERIES

Counselling Young People

Person-Centred Dialogues

Richard Bryant-Jefferies

Radcliffe Medical Press

Radcliffe Medical Press Ltd
18 Marcham Road
Abingdon
Oxon OX14 1AA
United Kingdom

www.radcliffe-oxford.com
The Radcliffe Medical Press electronic catalogue and online ordering facility.
Direct sales to anywhere in the world.

———————————————————————————

British Library Cataloguing in Publication Data

A catalogue record for this book is available from the British Library.

ISBN 1 85775 878 1

Typeset by Aarontype Limited, Easton, Bristol
Printed and bound by TJ International Ltd, Padstow, Cornwall

Contents

Foreword

I am delighted to contribute this Foreword to Richard's book. On the day that the script arrived I opened the envelope, deciding to just peruse the first few pages with the intention of dedicating a more appropriate time to read it later. This decision to just 'dip in' to the text was the undoing of all my rational thoughts about planning and organising my time! Needless to say, I was hooked in to the contents of this book immediately, from the opening paragraphs of the Preface!

Other than some years spent in an engineering training (following multiple school moves and failed O levels), my professional life has been substantially involved with working with young people, first as a youth worker in London, then as a teacher in Jamaica and for the last 25 years as a counsellor in higher education.

Richard has written a wonderfully creative and informative text here. I believe he has caught the subtlety of the person-centred therapeutic process extremely well while providing us with such engaging human stories played out through the dialogues between the young people, their counsellors and the counsellors' supervisors.

Richard has pointed out, appropriately, the importance of training and supervision for those taking on such therapeutic work with young people. Yet, at a personal level, in remembering my own experience, I do not underestimate the sheer impact of ideas and training experiences gained on quite modest weekend training courses while learning to be a part-time youth worker.

While studying to be a full-time youth worker, I came across some books by a particular author whose ideas I found resonated with my own view of the world. Indeed, these books were so influential upon me that I proceeded to base my whole professional way of being upon the ideas contained within them. It was only seven years later (having had five years as a full-time youth worker in London and a further two as a teacher in Jamaica), while preparing to embark upon a counselling training, that I returned to the essays I had written to discover that the author of these influential books had been Carl Rogers!

To me, Rogers' writings evoked a profound sense of humanity, of offering a way of being that had the potential to enhance the lives of others, and demonstrating a deep trustworthiness of human beings.

It is of no surprise to me that Rogers' ideas have permeated many fields of human interaction over the last 50 years (many of which are not recognised today as originating from the person-centred perspective) and, indeed, that

Rogers and his colleagues went far beyond the therapeutic relationship in their explorations of the potential these ideas held for human relating. The author has provided an excellent and concise description of the person-centred approach within his introduction. His later reference to more recent research (Everall and Paulson, 2002) on young people's views of helpful relationships indicates something of the enduring quality of Rogers' original ideas.

In the author's words, counsellors (and others working with young people) 'need to be able to adapt their style, to have a readiness and willingness to be open and to be psychologically alongside the young person'. The person-centred model of person-to-person relating provides a sound theoretical base for developing these skills and attributes. Richard comments on the importance of these relational components of the person-centred approach 'as a counter to the sense of isolation that frequently accompanies deep psychological and emotional problems, and the increase in [what he terms] a "rabid inauthenticity" within materialistic societies as we enter the 21st century'.

Richard has caught, wonderfully, in this text the sensitivity and delicacies of therapeutic interaction as well as the complex processes through which young people have to steer in their development towards adulthood. That young people today are under enormous pressures (commercial, relational, familial, etc.) is of little doubt. Indeed, a report by the Mental Health Foundation has noted that there is a clear consensus among those working in the field that there have been 'substantial increases in psychosocial disorders of youth since the Second World War in nearly all developed countries' (Mental Health Foundation, 1999).

In reading this text, I was aware of my sadness that, for many young people in our society, there may well not be a sufficiently human networked community within their fields of relating to enable their own development at times of crisis. The stories of Jodie and Nick and their experiences in the counselling process presented here provide the reader with an insight into the value of such developmental opportunities for young people.

In short, I am delighted to have been invited to contribute this Foreword to Richard's important and engaging text that combines, so elegantly, believable stories of young people with the provision of theoretical comment and developmental questions for the practitioner. I trust that this book will reach a wide audience of all those who are interested in and committed to the welfare and development of young people.

Colin Lago
**Formerly Director of the University of
Sheffield Counselling Service, 1987–2003
Now in independent practice as a counsellor,
supervisor, trainer and consultant**
October 2003

Foreword

What a treat it has been to read Richard Bryant-Jefferies' book! It has led me into a revisiting of my own years of counselling adolescents, and a reaffirmation of the deep conviction that the person-centred approach is powerfully effective with young people.

In the early 1980s, I was asked to work with large groups of students to counteract some of the bullying, drug use and alienation that earmarked the school culture during that period. A few colleagues and I would take 40 adolescents to residential retreats in the woods with barely any agenda except to try to live as a community. The students were selected by their own peers as 'group influencers' who they felt could speak for their clique. The groups which the participants influenced ranged from the drug users, to athletes, to outstanding scholars. Most did not have any established friendships in the new community and, at the outset, were belligerent and hostile toward others. In spite of all the threats their behaviour posed, we managed to remain person-centred, although insistent on certain areas of accountability.

Now this was a scary place to offer empathy and unconditional positive regard. I was warned over and over by the people who engaged my services that the person-centred approach was not applicable to young students. They needed to be controlled and led. As the following pages reveal, adolescents can be rejecting and cruel, and their behaviour is often outrageous. In hindsight though, I am sure that this approach was the *only* way for them to touch the depths to which they were able to go with one another. It was the ultimate trust in the capacity of those adolescents to reach into their humanity, and the congruence of the facilitators in wanting to form respectful relationships that cut through the shell of resistance that had hardened in authoritarian systems that oppress young people, their potential and their creativity. The outcomes of those communities were nothing short of miraculous.

This book goes a long way in explaining why the person-centred approach is so powerful with young people. It teases apart many of the fears, hurts, disappointments, familial problems and social assaults that encourage adolescents to close off, turn to drugs, attack others. After a clear and concise explanation of the theory, Richard takes us on two amazing journeys into the hearts and minds of Jodie and Nick – the clients described in the book. They are struggling with many of the obstacles in the path of most children trying to grow up in this period of social toxicity.

Each journey has three strands. The first strand belongs to the clients. Jodie and Nick begin to explore their experience, and gradually unravel some of the true feelings that are hampering their healthy development and eroding their human relationships. Their issues will be familiar to most of us, but the impact on, and the vulnerability of, the young client is so exquisitely expressed here that a reader cannot avoid being touched. As each one is heard and respected, rather than led or advised, the obstacles shift or even melt away, freeing them to become more self-accepting, move forward, and find more authentic connections with friends and family.

The counsellor's journeys provide the second strand within the two stories presented here. For readers who are presently practising or for those getting ready for practice, this book is a jewel! Unlike so many systems of counselling, the person-centred approach acknowledges how fully the practitioner is affected by the client, the relationship, the issues raised and the uncertainty about how to proceed. In *Counselling Young People: person-centred dialogues*, the reader will meet all the questions and quandaries around these issues, and recognise how subtle it is to maintain the values of the approach and relinquish power *over* the clients. If there is any doubt that growth in a counselling relationship occurs for the counsellor as well as the client, this book will dispel it.

The third strand is about supervision. Unlike many forms of supervision where the focus is on the client issues, person-centred supervision stays very much with the counsellor's experience and the situations that come up for them in their sessions. This is a place where the counsellor can face the anxieties about their work with clients, and the primal issues that are touched off in that work as well. The same values of respect, empathy and congruence are firmly held in these sessions. The meetings between counsellor and supervisor are very much a parallel of the client sessions.

Richard's creativity and compassion are apparent in this writing. He has created each of the characters, and each one touches the heart. My experience with adolescent clients has yielded much the same content as presented here, but rarely with more eloquence. The book is a real gift to anybody interested in raising or counselling young people; a marvellous *experience* of the person-centred approach for clients, counsellors and supervisors; and an illumination of the major tenets both theoretically and operationally.

Peggy Natiello PhD
Psychotherapist, educator, trainer, writer and consultant
in the person-centred approach
Arizona, USA
October 2003

Preface

Without doubt, counselling has become a growing feature in the lives of many young people. In schools, colleges, universities, within child and adolescent mental health services, within GP surgeries and social service centres, and through voluntary groups and charitable organisations, counsellors are being given an incredibly important role in helping children and young people cope with whatever has had, or is having, an adverse effect on them.

What do young people want most? To be given time. Space. Opportunity to make their own choices. Hope. Self-belief. To feel heard. For their needs to be taken seriously. To feel loved. The list can seem endless.

The issues that young people face extend across a multiplicity of difficult experiences: problems with best friends, bullying, sexual abuse, family difficulties, stress related to school work, fear of growing up, confusion and uncertainty about the future, loneliness – another seemingly endless list.

People – generally adults – say how kids don't need counselling, they need to get on with life. But young people today are not only put under enormous pressures, particularly commercial ones, but also emotional pressures with family break-up. The fashion industry exploits the senses of individuality and belonging; the record industry feeds on emotions and emerging sexuality; education emphasises knowledge at the expense of feelings; the quick-fix mentality rules – have now, pay later; keep high, don't drop; fast food, fast cars, fast drugs (and then the downers to slow them back down). There are a high number of teenage pregnancies; drug use is increasing and reaching into lower age groups; alcohol-related problems are rising.

Consumers in the making, there is a subtle, and sometimes not so subtle, conditioning that leaves young people convinced that the latest purchase will make them feel happy. And when they lose the happiness, when they're bored with it, they go and get something else to maintain the high. There is an emphasis on the external with little scope for exploration of inner space, of what it feels like to be a young person at the dawn of the twenty-first century. How do we empower young people to make healthy choices for themselves and emerge from the first two decades of their lives mentally, emotionally and physically prepared, with self-belief, sufficiently trusting of themselves and capable of clarity within their own natures, to move confidently into adulthood?

This book sets out to provide the reader with an experience of working with young people, and young people's issues, from a person-centred theoretical perspective. It aims to enable the reader to enter into the world of the young person and the counsellor who is working with them. It includes material to inform the training process of counsellors and many others who seek to work with young people. *Counselling Young People: person-centred dialogues* is intended as much for experienced counsellors as it is for trainees. It provides real insight into what can occur during counselling sessions, based on two settings: a youth counselling service and a secondary school. Reflections on the process and helpful summaries and points for discussion are included to stimulate further thought and debate.

Counselling Young People: person-centred dialogues will also be of value to the many healthcare and social care professionals who work with young people, along with educators and teachers. For all these professionals, the text demystifies what can occur in therapy, and at the same time provides useful ways of working that may be used by professionals other than counsellors.

I hope, as well, that this book will find its way into schools and into the material used for social learning.

Richard Bryant-Jefferies
October 2003

About the author

Richard Bryant-Jefferies qualified as a person-centred counsellor/therapist in 1994 and remains passionate about the application and effectiveness of this approach. Richard began working at a community drug and alcohol service in Surrey in early 1995. As well as offering counselling within this specialist arena, and establishing an alcohol counselling service within GP surgeries, he also supervised counsellors working with people with drug and alcohol problems. He has also worked as a general counsellor in a GP surgery. He continues to offer counselling supervision and workshops on alcohol-related themes. In the summer of 2003 Richard took up a sector management post for the Substance Misuse Service of Central and North West London Mental Health NHS Trust.

Richard had his first book on a counselling theme published in 2001, *Counselling the Person Beyond the Alcohol Problem* (Jessica Kingsley Publishers), providing theoretical yet practical insights into the application of the person-centred approach within the context of the 'cycle of change' model that has been widely adopted to describe the process of change in the field of addiction. Since then he has been writing for the *Living Therapy* series (Radcliffe Medical Press), producing an ongoing series of person-centred dialogues: *Problem Drinking*, *Time Limited Therapy in Primary Care*, *Counselling a Survivor of Child Sexual Abuse* and *Counselling a Recovering Drug User*. The aim of the series is to bring the reader a direct experience of the counselling process, an exposure to the thoughts and feelings of both client and counsellor as they encounter each other on the therapeutic journey.

In each of these books references are made as to how childhood experiences can and do affect an individual, leaving them with feelings about themselves that can have problematic effects later in life.

Richard is keen to bring the experience of the therapeutic process, from the standpoint and application of the person-centred approach, to a wider audience. He is convinced that the principles and attitudinal values of this approach and the emphasis it places on the therapeutic relationship are key to helping people create greater authenticity both in themselves and in their lives, leading to a fuller and more satisfying human experience.

Acknowledgements

In writing this book I would like to express my gratitude to the following professionals who contributed helpful and insightful feedback on the draft for this book:

Movena Lucas and Freda Noonan-Taylor, both of whom are clinical nurse specialists in NHS child and adolescent mental health services working with young people having drug and alcohol problems; and Emma Yates, a person-centred counsellor who specialises in working with young people in schools. They have all offered valuable comments concerning the content of the dialogue and the realism of what I have sought to portray.

Finally, I would also like to thank the series editor, Maggie Pettifer, for her continued encouragement towards the writing of the *Living Therapy* series. I know that she, like me, heartily believes in the significance of this style of presenting person-centred counselling applied to specific contexts and experiences.

Introduction

In many ways this book is probably unique insofar as it is written to offer the reader an opportunity to experience and to appreciate, through dialogue, some of the diverse and challenging issues that can arise when working with a young person who has had, and is struggling with, life in the teenage zone. It is composed of dialogues between fictitious clients and their counsellors, and between the counsellors and their supervisors. Within the dialogues are woven the reflective thoughts and feelings of the client, the counsellor and the supervisor.

The book has been written with the aim of demonstrating the counsellors' application of the person-centred approach (PCA) – a theoretical approach to counselling that has, at its heart, the power of the relational experience to offer the client an experience through which greater potential for authentic living may emerge – when working with young people. The approach is widely used by counsellors working in the UK today: in a membership survey in 2001 by the British Association for Counselling and Psychotherapy, 35.6 per cent of those responding claimed to work to the person-centred approach, while 25.4 per cent identified themselves as psychodynamic practitioners.

The reader may find it takes a while to adjust to the dialogue format. Many of the responses offered by the two counsellors, Sandy and Simon, are reflections of what their respective clients, Jodie and Nick, have said. This is not to be read as conveying a simple repetition of the client's words. Rather, the counsellor seeks to voice empathic responses, often with a sense of 'checking out' that they are hearing accurately what the client is saying. The client says something; the counsellor then conveys that they have heard it, sometimes with the same words, sometimes including a sense of what they feel may be being communicated through the client's tone of voice, facial expression, or simply the atmosphere of the moment. The client is then enabled to confirm that they have been heard accurately, or correct the counsellor in their perception. The client may then explore more deeply what they have been saying or move on, in either case with a sense that they have been heard and warmly accepted. To draw this to the reader's attention, I have attempted to highlight some of the reflections that occur throughout the work by inserting Sandy's and Simon's reflective thoughts in boxes throughout the dialogue.

The supervision sessions are included to offer the reader insight into the nature of therapeutic supervision in the context of the counselling profession, a method of supervising that I term 'collaborative review'. For many trainee counsellors, the use of supervision can be something of a mystery, and it is hoped that this book will go a long way to unravelling this. In the supervision sessions I seek to demonstrate the application of the supervisory relationship. My intention is to show how supervision of the counsellor is very much a part of the process of enabling a client to work through issues that are faced by young people in our society.

Many professions do not recognise the need for some form of personal and process supervision, and often what is offered is line management. However, counsellors are required to receive regular supervision in order to explore the dynamics of the relationship with the client, the impact of the work on the counsellor and on the client, to receive support, and to provide an opportunity for an experienced co-professional to monitor the supervisee's work in relation to ethical standards and codes of practice. The supervision sessions are included because they are an integral part of the therapeutic process. It is also hoped that they will help readers from other professions to recognise the value of some form of supportive and collaborative supervision in order to help them become more authentically present with their own clients.

I also favour an approach that is of a collaborative nature which I tend to describe as a process of 'collaborative review'. Merry (2002, p. 173) describes what he terms 'collaborative inquiry' as a 'form of research or inquiry in which two people (the supervisor and the counsellor) collaborate or co-operate in an effort to understand what is going on within the counselling relationship and within the counsellor'. There are, of course, as many models of supervision as there are models of counselling. In this book the supervisor is seeking to apply the attitudinal qualities of the person-centred approach.

It is the norm for all professionals working in the healthcare and social care environment in this age of regulation to be formally accredited or registered and to work to their own professional organisation's code of ethics or practice. For instance, registered counselling practitioners with the British Association for Counselling and Psychotherapy are required to have regular supervision and continuing professional development to maintain registration. While professionals other than counsellors will gain much from this book in their work with young people, it is essential that they follow the standards, safeguards and ethical codes of their own professional organisation, and are appropriately trained and supervised to work with their clients.

All characters in this book are fictitious and are not intended to bear resemblance to any particular person or persons.

The person-centred approach

The person-centred approach (PCA) was formulated by Carl Rogers, and references are made to his ideas within the text of the book. However, it will be helpful for readers who are unfamiliar with this way of working to have an appreciation of its theoretical base.

Rogers proposed that certain conditions, when present within a therapeutic relationship, would enable the client to develop towards what he termed 'fuller functionality'. Over a number of years he refined these ideas, which he defined as 'the necessary and sufficient conditions for constructive personality change'. These he described as follows:

1   Two persons are in psychological contact.
2   The first, whom we shall term the client, is in a state of incongruence, being vulnerable or anxious.
3   The second person, whom we shall term the therapist, is congruent or integrated in the relationship.
4   The therapist experiences unconditional positive regard for the client.
5   The therapist experiences an empathic understanding of the client's internal frame of reference and endeavours to communicate this experience to the client.
6   The communication to the client of the therapist's empathic understanding and unconditional positive regard is to a minimal degree achieved. (Rogers, 1957a, p. 6)

The first necessary and sufficient condition given for constructive personality change is that of 'two persons being in psychological contact'. However, although he later published this as simply 'contact' (Rogers, 1959), it is suggested (Wyatt and Sanders, 2002, p. 6) that this was actually written in 1953–54. They quote Rogers as defining contact in the following terms: 'Two persons are in psychological contact, or have the minimum essential relationship when each makes a perceived or subceived difference in the experiential field of the other' (Rogers, 1959, p. 207). A recent exploration of the nature of psychological contact from a person-centred perspective is given by Warner (2002).

Rogers defined empathy as meaning 'entering the private perceptual world of the other ... being sensitive, moment by moment, to the changing felt meanings which flow in this other person ... It means sensing meanings of which he or she is scarcely aware, but not trying to uncover totally unconscious feelings' (Rogers, 1980, p. 142). It is a very delicate process, and it provides, I believe, a foundation block. The counsellor's role is primarily to establish empathic rapport and communicate empathic understanding to the client.

Within this relationship the counsellor seeks to maintain an attitude of unconditional positive regard towards the client and all that they disclose. This is not 'agreeing with', it is simply warm acceptance. Rogers wrote, 'when the therapist is experiencing a positive, acceptant attitude towards whatever the client *is* at that moment, therapeutic movement or change is more likely to occur' (Rogers, 1980, p. 116). Mearns and Thorne suggest that 'unconditional positive regard is the label given to the fundamental attitude of the person-centred counsellor towards her client. The counsellor who holds this attitude deeply values the humanity of her client and is not deflected in that valuing by any particular client behaviours. The attitude manifests itself in the counsellor's consistent acceptance of and enduring warmth towards her client' (Mearns and Thorne, 1988, p. 59).

Last, but by no means least, is the state of being that Rogers referred to as congruence, but which has also been described in terms of 'realness', 'transparency', 'genuineness', 'authenticity'. Indeed, Rogers wrote that '... genuineness, realness or congruence ... this means that the therapist is openly being the feelings and attitudes that are flowing within at the moment ... the term transparent catches the flavour of this condition'. Putting this into the therapeutic setting, we can say that 'congruence is the state of being of the counsellor when her outward responses to her client consistently match the inner feelings and sensations which she has in relation to her client' (Mearns and Thorne, 1999, p. 84).

I would suggest that any congruent expression by the counsellor of their feelings or reactions has to emerge through the process of being in therapeutic relationship with the client. It is a disciplined response and not an open door to endless self-disclosure. Congruent expression is perhaps most appropriate and therapeutically valuable where it is informed by the existence of an empathic understanding of the client's inner world, and is offered in a climate of a genuine warm acceptance towards the client.

PCA regards the relationship that we have with our clients, and the attitude that we hold within that relationship, to be key factors. In my experience, many adult psychological difficulties develop out of life experiences that involve problematic, conditional or abusive relational experiences. This can be centred in childhood or later in life. What is important is that the individual is left, through relationships that have a negative conditioning effect, with a distorted perception of themselves and their potential as a person. I see many people who have learned from childhood experience beliefs such as 'I can never be good enough to be praised for what I have achieved; I never match my parents' expectations' or 'No one was ever there for me when I was hurting; perhaps I am unlovable'. The result is a loss of a positive sense of self, and the individual adapts to maintain the newly learned concept of self. This is then lived out, possibly throughout life, with the person seeking to satisfy what they have come to believe about themselves: being unable to achieve, feeling unable or undeserving to be loved, though perhaps in both cases maintaining a constant desperation to receive what they never had. Yet, perversely, they may then sabotage any possibility of gaining what they want in order to maintain the negatively conditioned sense of self and the sense of satisfaction that this gives them because they have developed such a strong identity with it.

It is my belief that by offering someone a non-judgemental, warm, accepting and authentic relationship, the person can grow into a fresh sense of self in which their potential as a person can become more fulfilled. Such an experience fosters an opportunity for the client to redefine themselves as they experience the presence of the therapist's congruence, empathy and unconditional positive regard. This process can take time. Often the personality change that is required to sustain a shift away from what have been termed 'conditions of worth' requires a lengthy period of therapeutic work, bearing in mind that the person may be struggling to unravel a sense of self that has been developed, sustained and reinforced for many decades of life.

The term 'conditions of worth' applies to the conditioning that is frequently present in childhood, and at other times in life, when a person experiences that their worth is conditional on their doing something, or behaving, in a certain way. This is usually to satisfy someone else's needs, and can be contrary to the client's own sense of what would be a satisfying experience. The values of others become a feature of the individual's structure of self. The person moves away from being true to themselves, learning instead to remain 'true' to their conditioned sense of worth. This state of being in the client is challenged by the person-centred therapist offering them unconditional positive regard and warm acceptance. Such a therapist, by genuinely offering these therapeutic attitudes, provides the client with an opportunity to be exposed to what may be a new experience or one that in the past they have dismissed, preferring to stay with that which matches and therefore reinforces their conditioned sense of worth and sense of self. Unconditional positive regard and warm acceptance offered consistently over time can, and does, enable clients to begin to question their beliefs about themselves and to begin to build into their structure of self the capacity to see and experience themselves as being of value for who they are. It enables them to liberate themselves from the constraints of patterns of conditioning.

A crucial feature or factor in this process is the presence of what Rogers termed 'the actualizing tendency', a tendency towards fuller and more complete personhood with an associated greater fulfilment of their potentialities. The role of the person-centred counsellor is to provide the facilitative climate within which this tendency can work constructively. The 'therapist trusts the actualizing tendency of the client and truly believes that the client who experiences the freedom of a fostering psychological climate will resolve his or her own problems' (Bozarth, 1998, p. 4). This is fundamental to the application of the person-centred approach. Rogers (1986, p. 198) wrote: 'the person-centred approach is built on a basic trust in the person ... (It) depends on the actualizing tendency present in every living organism – the tendency to grow, to develop, to realize its full potential. This way of being trusts the constructive directional flow of the human being towards a more complex and complete development. It is this directional flow that we aim to release.'

The therapeutic relationship is central. A therapeutic approach such as person-centred affirms that it is not what you do so much as 'how you are' with your client that is therapeutically significant, and this 'how you are' has to be received by the client. Gaylin (2001, p. 103) highlights the importance of client perception. 'If clients believe that their therapist is working on their behalf – if they perceive caring and understanding – then therapy is likely to be successful. It is the condition of attachment and the perception of connection that have the power to release the faltered actualization of the self.' He goes on to stress how 'we all need to feel connected, prized – loved', describing human beings as 'a species born into mutual interdependence', and that there 'can be no self outside the context of others'. He highlights that 'loneliness is dehumanizing and isolation anathema to the human condition. The relationship,' he suggests, 'is what psychotherapy is all about.'

There is currently growing interest in, and much debate about, theoretical developments within the person-centred world and its application. Discussions on the theme of Rogers' therapeutic conditions presented by various key members of the person-centred community have recently been published (Bozarth and Wilkins, 2001; Haugh and Merry 2001; Wyatt, 2001; Wyatt and Sanders, 2002). It seems to me that the relational component of the person-centred approach, based on the presence of the core conditions, is emerging strongly as a counter to the sense of isolation that frequently accompanies deep psychological and emotional problems, and the increase in what I would term a 'rabid inauthenticity' within materialistic societies as we enter the twenty-first century.

This is obviously a very brief introduction to the approach. Person-centred theory continues to develop as practitioners and theoreticians consider its application in various fields of therapeutic work and extend our theoretical understanding of developmental and therapeutic processes. At times it feels like it has become more than just individuals; rather it feels like a group of colleagues, based around the world, working together to penetrate deeper towards a more complete theory of the human condition. It is an exciting time.

Counselling young people

Counselling young people is becoming more widespread in our society. Since the 1960s, counselling has become more of a feature in schools, and youth counselling services have become established both in the voluntary and statutory sectors of health and social care. With this have come the many challenges associated with forming a therapeutic relationship with young people, and the seemingly difficult legal landscape associated with the young person's right to confidentiality and their competence to consent to treatment. The legal position has recently been usefully discussed by Jenkins (2002), who argues the need for counsellors and psychotherapists working with children and young people to be familiar with the background to the establishment of the Gillick principle and the ensuing case law. It is not the intention in this volume to explore this; the reader is, however, encouraged to undertake their own research on this topic.

Let us turn to the therapeutic relationship with young people. What are the factors that contribute to a successful therapeutic experience? From a recent piece of research into adolescent perspectives on the therapeutic alliance, it has been suggested that the factors of 'therapeutic environment . . . the climate or "ambience" within which the therapist and client functioned which set the tone for what was to follow'; 'the uniqueness of the therapeutic relationship . . . comprised of an egalitarian foundation, a sense of trust and respect, and a view that the therapist was a special friend'; and certain 'therapist chacteristics . . . a sense that the therapist was authentic, open and sincerely cared . . . manifested through a genuine emotional response that was described as sensitive, sympathetic and kind' are of primary importance (Everall and Paulson, 2002, pp. 81–3). These attitudinal qualities bear a close resemblance to those posited by Rogers as fundamental conditions for constructive personality change. Indeed the authors of this study comment that 'the development of a therapeutic alliance with adolescents appears to be consistent with the research on the therapeutic triad of empathy, genuineness and respect (Rogers, 1957a). Warmth and empathy were clearly identified by our participants who used identical words that Rogers used to identify the core conditions' (Everall and Paulson, 2002, pp. 84–5).

However, the study also highlighted negative experiences, and these the adolescents referred to in terms of the relationship with the therapist 'being similar to other interactions with adults in terms of a power differential and was identified as having an authoritarian foundation'. The negative impact of the therapist taking the role of 'expert', of not listening to what the young person was saying about their experiences, and the feeling that they were not being treated respectfully were highlighted. In particular, the authors of the study report, 'lack of respect resulted in withdrawal from engagement' (Everall and Paulson, 2002, p. 85).

The fact that the young people saw the counselling relationship as 'special', and the therapist as 'a special friend', offers valuable insight into the inner world of the young clients. They indicated how important this was, and what a contrast it was to their usual experience of being in relationship with adults. This contrast was reported as being difficult at first – the client perhaps being wary, not sure what was going on, finding their expectations challenged and taking time to settle into a feeling of trust towards the therapist.

It seems highly likely that for effective counselling of young people there needs to be an adaptation in style, a readiness and willingness by the counsellor to be open, to really want to be psychologically alongside the young person, to enable that young person to feel at ease and to share whatever is present for them. I have certainly come across counsellors who participate in other activities with the client, chatting with them as they do so, encouraging the client to share in a more conversational form of therapeutic encounter.

This is not a licence for anything goes. The therapist remains disciplined, but open to the means of communication that most effectively help them build a therapeutic alliance with the client. For the person-centred counsellor, the intention will be to be open to direction from the client, to be prepared to learn what most helps that young person gain what they need from the therapeutic experience.

Gaylin highlights the particular importance of therapist congruence when working with young people. He suggests that 'before they entrust adults with their deeply personal thoughts and feelings they need to believe the adults are worthy of that trust. Children are masters of nonverbal communication – more so than adults – and thus can sense deception and guile. Simply put, young people of all ages demand congruence in their therapists if therapy is to be effective' (Gaylin, 2001, p. 124). I would suggest that as adults are honest with young people genuinely – and authentically, with clear self-awareness and openness to their own experiencing – then there is a much higher likelihood that young people will feel encouraged to become more real themselves, more openly present and able to engage more fully, and with clarity of awareness, with the range of experiencing that is open to them as human beings.

Person-centred theory and education

While this volume is not written to address the application of the person-centred approach within education, it is worth briefly acknowledging that Carl Rogers addressed this theme both in his books and in various papers and lectures (Rogers, 1957b, 1967, 1969, 1977, 1980). The attitudinal values of the person-centred approach, while having therapeutic application, actually extend beyond that into all situations in which people are required to work together, where the forming of human relationships is a crucial part of a particular endeavour.

Rogers wrote of the notion of 'whole-person learning' (1980), which encompasses both feelings and ideas. Indeed, he regarded it as requiring a merging of the two approaches, a bringing together of 'cognitive learning, which has always been needed, and affective-experiential learning, which is so underplayed in education today' (1980, p. 264). He goes on to define 'what it means to learn as a whole person' as involving 'learning of a *unified* sort, at the cognitive, feeling and gut levels, with a clear *awareness* of the different aspects of this unified learning' (1980, p. 266).

He comments on how schooling has stressed the cognitive, teaching from the neck up, which he regarded as a way of avoiding any feeling connected with learning. As a result, he argued, while we may know intellectual facts, we become removed from feeling our knowledge. This split he regarded as extremely damaging and, added to this, he suggested that it meant that the excitement had gone out of learning.

In today's exam-centred schooling I wonder what he would be thinking, and feeling! Do young people today feel excited by their learning? Or are the main feelings present those of anxiety linked to the next exam or statutory testing, or emptiness because lessons may have a significant tendency to prepare young people for exams and not for the wonder of life, which is where the real excitement is.

Rogers' 'necessary and sufficient conditions for constructive personality change' (1957a) have wide application; indeed he argued that when these attitudinal conditions are present they 'would promote any whole person learning – that they would hold for the classroom as well as the therapist's office' (Rogers, 1980, p. 270). He then goes on to outline the application of these attitudinal conditions in the context of the learning environment.

For the teacher, or 'facilitator of learning', he argued that 'when the facilitator is a real person, being what he or she is, entering into relationship with the learners without presenting a front or a façade, the facilitator is much more likely to be effective' (Rogers, 1980, p. 271). He emphasises the importance of the teacher being able to experience their feelings, to live and be them, and communicate them if appropriate. The teacher becomes authentically present and is therefore enabled to engage in a genuine person-to-person encounter with those who are learning.

Rogers highlighted too the importance of 'prizing, acceptance and trust', a willingness to accept the worth of each individual, to prize them as the unique person that they are and trust in each young person's capacity and potential as human beings. This acceptance should extend to a student's 'occasional apathy, their erratic desires to explore by-roads of knowledge, as well as their disciplined efforts to achieve major goals' (Rogers, 1980, pp. 271–2).

He also outlines the importance of 'empathic understanding' as 'a further element that establishes a climate for self-initiated experiential learning' (Rogers, 1980, p. 272). This involves the teacher being able to appreciate the experience of learning from the student's perspective, of standing in their shoes, helping their view to feel validated and understood, rather than 'judged or evaluated'.

However, none of these attitudinal conditions matter if they are not experienced by the student as being present within the teacher. Of course, young people at school are likely to be suspicious at first, but Rogers goes on to give examples of how the application of the attitudinal elements can and does make a positive contribution to the learning process.

Rogers cites a number of research papers to support his conclusion that these interpersonal conditions are 'significantly and positively related' to a number of educational outcomes: 'greater gain in reading achievement (Aspy, 1965); grade point average (Pierce, 1966); cognitive growth (Aspy, 1967, 1969; Aspy and Hadlock, 1967); an increase in creative interest and productivity (Moon, 1966); levels of cognitive thinking and to the amount of student-initiated talk (Aspy and Roebuck, 1970) ... the student's better utilization of their abilities and greater confidence in themselves (Schmuck, 1966)' (Rogers, 1980, pp. 277–8).

The person-centred approach has wide application as a way of being that can encourage people, including young people, to become more authentically present. Rogers wrote, in terms of the effects of 'being in relationship with an effective therapist', that 'the client begins to realize: "I am not compelled to be simply the creation of others, molded by their expectancies, shaped by their demands. I am not compelled to be a victim of unknown forces in myself. I am less and less a creature of influences in myself which operate beyond my ken in the realms of the unconscious. I am increasingly the architect of self. I am free to will and choose. I can, through accepting my individuality, my 'isness,' become more of my uniqueness, more of my potentiality"' (Rogers, 1963, pp. 48–9).

Surely a goal of education is to prepare the young person for this possibility?

PART I

Counselling a young person in a youth counselling setting

Setting the scene

Sandy works for a youth counselling service which is based in a local YMCA. The service had a policy of fast-tracking young people where drugs were known to be involved. She has been working there for three years, and finds it very rewarding working with young people. She also works in other settings and has a small private practice.

Referrals are from various sources as well as self-referral. She enjoys the wide range of issues that her clients bring. The referral for Jodie had come from her mother. They had written back and said that they wanted confirmation from Jodie that she wanted to come. She had called and left a message, although it wasn't very enthusiastic, so she was expecting her to be brought by an exasperated parent to be 'sorted out'. She knew that there were drugs involved, and she was OK with that. She had done a placement in her training with a drug team and had attended drug awareness training sessions. It had really opened her eyes. And it was by no means an uncommon issue among the young people that she saw.

She wasn't limited to any number of sessions with the young people that she saw, and she was grateful for that. She knew of other services that were not so fortunate.

Sandy is 38, not in a relationship, having gone through divorce five years previously, one of the results of the effect of her counselling training. It had marked a real change in her life, an expansion of her interests and a change of career. She had previously worked in a large departmental store. But that seemed a long time ago, almost a past life, if you believe in that possibility.

So she waited for her new client, Jodie, to arrive. It was always an apprehensive time, but she knew she was excited too. She believed passionately in the effectiveness of the person-centred approach and was looking forward to working towards forming a therapeutic relationship with Jodie.

CHAPTER 1

Counselling session 1: first contact – the counsellor keeps it low key

Sandy began the session by commenting on the nature of confidentiality and its limits, and the fact that there was no limit to the number of sessions; that was something they could decide on as they went along.

'Yeah, that's cool,' had been Jodie's response. She then lapsed into silence.

Sandy also mentioned that they had up to 50 minutes, but it was really up to Jodie to decide how much time she wanted, and how she wanted to use the time.

Throughout all that Sandy had said, Jodie had sat looking slightly to the side of Sandy, avoiding eye contact. She spoke, and as she did so shifted her focus. 'Didn't want to come today.' Jodie now sat staring somewhat defiantly back at Sandy, her counsellor.

'You look pretty angry at having to come at all.'

'Yeah. My mum, she insisted I come. What does she know?'

'What does she know?'

'Not a lot.'

Jodie lapsed into silence. She really didn't want to be there. Wanted to be out with her mates, up the town, hanging out, checking out the lads. Chilling out and having a few laughs.

'So your mum knows not a lot and you really don't want to be here, Jodie.' Sandy sought to keep a focus on what Jodie had been saying, wanting her to feel heard, wanting to encourage her to feel listened to.

Jodie continued to sit and stare.

'Pretty defiant, huh?'

Jodie didn't reply. She was thinking of Mac, her ex-boyfriend – they hadn't actually met up much, most of the time they had texted each other. But he was history. Nice bum though . . .

Sandy continued to sit and wait. She wasn't fazed by Jodie's attitude. She fully accepted that Jodie had good reason to be the way that she was. She wanted her to feel quite accepted. She could sense that Jodie was very much with her own thoughts.

> Offering warm acceptance is an important aspect of person-centred counsel-
> ling. Jodie is being how she needs to be. That needs to be accepted. Right
> from the start of the counselling encounter, the person-centred counsellor
> is seeking to offer a therapeutic climate. Sandy is allowing her to be and not
> seeking to disturb that. She is attentive as well to her own body language
> and facial expression, seeking to convey openness to Jodie.

'So, feel free to say anything you want to say, and feel free to say nothing. It's up
to you. And I really hope that I can be helped to understand whatever may be
troubling you.' She spoke authentically. This was what she hoped and she
wanted to communicate it to her new client.

Typical bloody counsellor, Jodie thought, not that she knew what a typical
bloody counsellor was, but it sounded the kind of nice sort of thing that she
thought counsellors said, to make you like them, to make you trust them.
She didn't trust anyone, and she wasn't going to trust this woman sitting opposite her. She decided to say nothing and the silence continued.

Sandy only had Jodie's body language to empathise with, and she was sitting
somewhat slumped in the chair, but she didn't look relaxed. Much more preoccupied with her own thoughts. She began to look at her nails, rubbing the
tips as if to somehow make them smoother. She had a kind of plum-coloured
nail varnish, looked like it had been on for a few days, bit cracked round the
edges. She had some like it herself at home. Sandy took in the young girl sitting
before her. Her hair was quite long and dark, well past her shoulders. She
would brush it away from her forehead every now and then, turning her head
to one side as she did so. It was quite a dramatic movement in many ways.
Her lipstick sort of matched her nails, well, nearly, but it was just a tad too pink.
Sandy pulled herself out of her thoughts, realising that she wasn't really focusing on Jodie, but had begun to sink into her own thoughts, speculations and,
well, judgements.

'I was just sitting here like you, looking at your nails. Good colour that, got some
myself at home.'

The counsellor seeks to connect with the client, offering something of herself. She wants to offer the opportunity of dialogue with the client. She knows from experience that she could sit here throughout the hour without the client saying anything, and maybe there is a place for that with adults, but with a young person, aged 15, it felt more appropriate to try and encourage communication. Of course, the client is communicating silence, although it is a silence with attitude. Young people can find counselling really strange. Being faced with an adult can bring up all kinds of reactions and assumptions that may need to be overcome. Also, the nature of the actual interactions can seem odd at first.

Sandy does not speak out of a sense of anxiety. She is speaking from a wish to connect with Jodie, to find some way to help her to engage in the process. In reality, the process has already started. Silence and an attitude of not wanting to be there.

'Oh yeah.' Jodie continued to look at her own nails.

'Yeah. Got it at . . . ,' she thought, 'actually I'm not sure. Can spend hours getting them right, can't you?'

Jodie blew out a short breath through her nose, making a kind of derisory sound. 'Try telling my mum that.'

'Your mum? Doesn't understand . . .' Sandy didn't manage to finish what she was saying, being interrupted by Jodie, who had moved in the chair, turning herself and slumping back down again, continuing to stare at her nails. She heard her take a deep breath and blow it back out heavily.

'Mums, huh?'

'Yeah.' Jodie didn't say any more; she still stared at her nails. She wondered if she could go yet, but guessed probably not. But she thought she'd try it. 'Can I go now?'

'If that's what you really want to do.'

Jodie swept her hair to one side again; it had fallen back across her face. 'You're just saying that.'

'Well, I am saying it, and I do mean it. If you want to go, if you want to be somewhere else, then, yeah, go for it. But if you do go, do you want to come back another time? I'd be happy to see you again. Sitting here like this can feel so unreal sometimes, hard to get used to. But I'd be happy to see you again.'

Jodie sort of went to get up, but stopped; something had stopped her but she didn't know what. She had wanted to go, but somehow she was still sitting there. She wasn't sure why.

'It's really weird, sitting here, I mean, I don't know what to say, you know?'

'Yeah, it is weird, and I do it every day and sometimes I don't know what to say either.'

Jodie looked up. 'You should know what to say. You're the counsellor.'

'Maybe, but I still don't always know what to say.'

'Oh.' Jodie went back to her visual examination of her plum nails.

Another silence. It was broken by Jodie. 'I'm just fed up.'

'Just fed up?' Sandy emphasised the 'just' in her response.

'Yeah. It's like, I don't know, it's like I can never get anything right. People always on my back. Always telling me what to do, what's good for me. The fuck do they know.'

'That can be tough, people always on at you.'

Jodie nodded.

Sandy felt a little more sense of connection to Jodie. She knew she needed to take it slowly and stay with her, but at the same time be true to herself as well. No point in trying to be what I'm not, she thought.

'It's mum, she doesn't like me going out so much, gives me grief.' She shook her head. 'Fucking nightmare.'

'Mhmm, fucking nightmare.' Sandy dropped the tone of her voice as she spoke, allowing Jodie to reflect further on her feelings.

That was a surprise. Sandy didn't look the kind of person who said 'fuck'.

'She doesn't understand.'

'Mhmm. They never do.' Shit, thought Sandy, that was me and my mother, not Jodie and hers. 'Yours doesn't understand you, neither did mine.'

Jodie tossed her head back slightly. Who cares about your mum, that's your problem, she thought to herself. And yet part of her also felt a kind of . . . she didn't know how to describe the feeling, but it kind of felt like there was some kind of link, some sort of, yeah, sort of being somehow on the same side. Then the part of her that didn't give a damn about what Sandy had experienced reasserted itself. 'Don't suppose yours was anything like mine.'

'Probably not. Everyone's different.'

'Yeah, mine's different all right, fucking nightmare. Does my head in. Does my fucking head in.'

Sandy nodded. 'Yeah, does your head in, Jodie, does your fucking head in.'

Jodie felt herself smile but she tried to keep it to herself. She didn't really want Sandy to see it. It was her smile, but it wasn't important, and she didn't want it seen. She didn't want to smile, she wanted to feel pissed off. She liked feeling pissed off.

'Just goes on at me, all the time, don't wear that, don't like you being with whoever, why can't you help around the house, what do you do all day, always wanting money. Nag, nag, nag.'

'Mhmm.'

'She doesn't let up. Now she's really having a go, since she found the dope. Snooping round my room. Fuck it. And she brings me here, wants you to sort me out. "They'll tell you." ' She paused, before continuing. 'Shit, I'm 15, I want a life.'

'Yeah, I really hear how important that is, you want a life.' Sandy stayed with where Jodie had got to, deciding not to take her back to the dope. She didn't want the session to become dope-centred, though she was going to ensure that Jodie was aware that she had heard her mention it.

While Sandy has knowledge about dope (cannabis) she is not going to allow the session to become 'substance-centred'. Here, Sandy is seeking to build a relationship with Jodie. She wants to encourage Jodie to speak freely, to build a rapport with her. She didn't want to jump in and start making judgements or giving advice. So, Jodie had some dope in her room. Lots of young people do. If she came on heavy about it, well, Jodie'd very likely walk out. What good would that serve? No, she wanted to place the emphasis on building a therapeutic relationship.

'Yeah.'

'And you smoke a bit of dope.'

Jodie nodded. 'Nothing wrong in that, is there? Everyone does.'

'Doesn't feel wrong to you?'

'No. I like it. Makes me feel good, yeah, takes the edge off everything, yeah, it's cool. Yeah. And it gives me a bit of peace.'

'So it gives you a lot of things, yeah?'

'Yeah.' Jodie was nodding. 'Just like feeling kinda mellow, you know, yeah, nicely cool, with a little bit of sharpness too. Kind of makes my music sound better.'

'That's a good feeling. Nicely cool but a good effect on music.'

'You ever smoked?'

'Uh-hu.'

Big question. Sandy gives an honest response. She hasn't gone into detail, didn't get a chance to as Jodie responded quickly. How much does a counsellor self-disclose? Could the setting affect how much a counsellor self-discloses? Maybe Sandy is more open because of her experience of working on placement at a substance misuse service. Maybe, maybe not.

'So you're not gonna be able to tell me to stop.'

'I'm not here to tell you to stop.'

'What are you here for then?'

'To listen, to give you time and space to talk, to be real with you and hopefully you will be real with me.' Sandy spoke genuinely. She didn't see any point in speaking in any other way.

'But you're not gonna tell me to stop.'

'No, what good would that do anyway?'

'Not a lot.'

'Well then. So you smoke a bit of dope. I can give you some information about it, what effects it has and stuff, got some new leaflets come through, info on all kinds of stuff.'

'Yeah, such as?'

'Pretty much everything. And stuff on overdose as well.'
'That sounds scary. I only smoke a bit of puff.'

Puff and dope are some of the names used for cannabis.

'Yeah, it is scary, and you aren't going to overdose on puff, but you can on other substances.'
'Yeah? Don't know much about that. Don't think I want to know.'
'OK, up to you, but the leaflets are here if you want them. There's one for parents too.'
'That's a good idea. Don't suppose she'll read it but . . . Worth taking, I suppose.'
'You don't sound too hopeful.' Sandy was touched by the hint of resignation in Jodie's voice. It sounded like she was replaying something that had occurred many times before.
'She doesn't listen to me. Never has.'
'That's tough, not feeling listened to, yeah?'

Sandy offers a simple but questioning response, seeking to acknowledge the feelings associated with just how tough it can be.

Jodie nodded, and she sighed.
Sandy matched her behaviour with a sigh, and added, 'Sums it up, huh?'
Jodie was back looking at her nails again. She'd been over it so many times with her mother, who never listened, always had to have the final say, always had to have it her way. And she, Jodie, was pissed off with it. She didn't say anything. What was the point? Nothing was going to change. What-was-the-point.
'I think I want to go now.'
'OK, would you like to come back?'
'I don't know. Maybe, but on my own. I don't want my mother hovering around outside, waiting to pounce on me and ask all kinds of questions.'
'Mhmm, that sounds pretty reasonable to me. Next week OK, same time, same day?'
Jodie nodded. 'Yeah, OK. I'll see you then.'
'Before you go, I do want to remind you that what you say here is confidential, we won't speak to your mother. We only break confidentiality, as I said earlier, if you are threatening serious harm to yourself, or someone else, or if you disclose anything connected with child abuse. So, if your mum should phone up, we won't be telling her anything. This is your time, your space, and you can use it as you want, talk about what you want, whatever.'
That's good to hear, Jodie thought as she got up. Never get much of my own space at home. 'Thanks.' She picked up the leaflets and headed out the door, no doubt to be pounced upon by a waiting parent.

> Jodie has already heard this, but she was in another place and clearly hadn't really heard it in the way that she now has. So something has changed, even though it was a short session. Jodie has been allowed to make her own choice. She has not been formally assessed. Sandy, and the culture of the organisation, is concerned with building relationships with clients and trying to help them feel accepted so that they may choose to engage with the service.

Jodie left and immediately got questioned. Had the counsellor told her to stop? What was she going to do about it? Jodie ignored her mother, then gave her the drug leaflet for parents.

'Read this.'

'Have you made another appointment?'

'Yes, and I want to come on my own next time.'

There then ensued a heated discussion as to whether Jodie would actually come to the session, which ended with Jodie saying she was fed up never feeling trusted, that at times it just made her feel like doing exactly what she was being told was expected of her. She was going to attend, if only to prove her mother wrong.

Meanwhile, Sandy sat and pondered the session. She felt that at least she had managed to gain some connection with Jodie, that they had had what felt like meaningful contact. She thought that she had listened and given Jodie space. She recognised that this was probably a really odd experience for her, and that she might take time to get used to it. But that was OK.

> It is early days. It takes time for a therapeutic relationship to develop. Jodie has never had counselling before and is no doubt distrustful of adults. She will have come with expectations probably of being told what to do. She didn't experience this and now she has to find her own way of making sense of it. She knows the door is open for her to come back to, if she wants to. What a way to start her summer break.
>
> Part of her really didn't see much point to counselling, but it gave her a break from stuff, maybe it would keep her mother happy – and that was a real bonus – but she really needed to come on her own. She wanted her own space, her own time.
>
> She thought about Sandy. She wasn't sure how old she was. She didn't kind of feel as old as she looked, somehow. The more she thought about Sandy, the more she found herself remembering bits of the session. Yeah, it had felt good to talk, though she hadn't really said much. She looked at the clock. Shit! She was meeting up with her mates over by the supermarket in 30 minutes, and she had to get herself ready.

Points for discussion

- How would you have felt sitting opposite Jodie defiantly affirming that she didn't want to be there?
- How effective is Sandy in building a relationship with Jodie?
- Was she right to let Jodie go?
- What might have been the result of Sandy talking at length about the dangers of cannabis use?
- If Sandy had taken a lengthy history from Jodie of her life and family, would that have been likely to have encouraged her to continue coming, or put her off?
- Write your own notes for the session.

CHAPTER 2

Counselling session 2: getting focused, becoming angry, finding calm

Jodie arrived. OK, she was ten minutes late, but she just hadn't got herself ready in time. Because the counselling service was quite close to where she lived – only a short bus ride – it was easy for her to get to. And besides, she'd arranged to meet up with friends afterwards. She'd told them the next day. They thought it was really cool having a counsellor, but thought it funny that her mother was so worried about her smoking dope.

'Come on, Jode, it's what we all do.'

'Yeah. I'm not planning to stop, but if it keeps my mum happy for me to go along, then that's what I'm gonna do for a while anyway. But I'll stop smoking at home, that was bad news.'

'Yeah, well, we don't have to go home, we can go up the park anytime, it's nice, it's warm.'

'Yeah, course we can.' The three of them linked arms and headed off to the park. Ally, Emma and Jodie – been friends for a few years now. Did everything together. Yeah, anything for a laugh.

Jodie had been thinking back to that conversation when she heard Sandy call her name. She didn't reply, just trudged down the corridor to the counselling room.

'Hi.' Sandy smiled at her. 'Good to see you again.' She genuinely felt pleased to see Jodie. It couldn't have been easy for her to come back. Young people could be so busy, hectic social lives, own agendas. So, yes, she felt good that she had come back and she acknowledged to herself that she was kind of curious as to why.

'Keeps my mum off my case.' Sandy was looking around the room as she spoke.

'That why you came back, to keep her off your case?'

Jodie nodded. 'Yeah. Friends think it's funny.'

'You've told your friends about coming here then.'

'They kind of think it's funny me coming here. I suppose I do too.'

Jodie has said 'funny' twice now. Sandy did not empathise with it the first time, so maybe Jodie wants her to hear it, hence her saying it again.

'Funny – for them and for you?'

'Yeah, guess so. Don't know what to talk about though.'

'Can be hard to think of something to say, sometimes.'

'Well, you know what I think about my mum.' Jodie sighed. 'I just get so pissed off sometimes, you know, just, I dunno, just feel I don't know what I feel . . . I get so angry. She hates that. But I feel really good. Great buzz. Yeah, really like it. Gets you respect too, you know. People don't mess with me much, not at school. We got a reputation to keep.'

'We . . .?'

'Me and Em and Ally. Been together for a long while now, years, brought up together, live not exactly in the same street but pretty close. Yeah, we really get on well, do what we want, have a few laughs, mess around.'

'Sounds like they are really important to you.'

'More than anyone in the whole world. Nothing comes between us, nothing. Yeah, they're cool.'

'Uhuh, you kind of stand together, nothing, no one comes between you.'

'Not even boys!' Jodie smiled and looked up at Sandy.

'Not even boys, yeah, you are close.'

They both ended up smiling and Jodie was suddenly aware of just how good it felt, to be sitting here, talking, smiling, it felt good. What the hell was happening to her? It didn't feel right. It felt good, but it suddenly didn't feel comfortable, felt wrong. She looked down again and said nothing.

Sandy had noticed the sudden change and although she had no idea what it was about she did feel that it was communicating something to her. Should she empathise with the body language? She realised she was deliberating in her own mind and the moment had passed.

Sandy loses her spontaneity. She does not know why. Another time, another client, she may have responded by saying something like, 'Uncomfortable?'

Sandy decided to say something, to remind Jodie that she could use the time, her time, however she needed to. 'So, anything in particular you want to say, or check out, try and make sense of?'

Jodie shook her head and continued to stare into the space ahead of her. She wasn't thinking about anything, no, just staring, blank, nothing. She just sat, and time passed.

After a few minutes Sandy was thinking to herself that, well, if Jodie wanted to use the time this way, then maybe she was getting something from it, but her expression, the way she was slumped in the chair, she just looked totally out of it. It crossed her mind as to whether she might have smoked some dope before the session. She decided to raise the fact that she didn't feel particularly connected to Jodie. She felt that being real with her might be helpful.

'I feel really cut off from you, Jodie, like you've gone into a place in yourself that I can't reach.' The words Sandy spoke reflected how she felt. Jodie just seemed to be 'over there', out of reach. Sandy also wanted to say it in a way that reflected her sense of responsibility for reaching out to her client.

Jodie heard Sandy and shifted a little in the chair, but still said nothing.

Sandy could feel frustration rising in her, and she was surprised by this. It wasn't something she often felt with clients, but there was something about Jodie's mannerism, her unwillingness to respond ... Sandy was used to working with people in silence: sometimes it was a 'working silence', at other times very much an 'uncomfortable silence'. But this didn't seem to be either. The thought came into her head that it was more of an 'empty silence'. She did a reality check on herself. How was she feeling? Yes, there was a sense of emptiness present for her, but she was not at all clear as to where it had come from. Could it be connected to Jodie, what she might be experiencing? She couldn't be sure, but it was very present and very persistent.

Sandy realised that she was fast becoming overly absorbed in her own reactions and forgetting Jodie. She looked across at Jodie as she sat there, slumped down in the chair, looking at her nails again like she had last week, looking really intense and yet somehow she felt like a shell. She couldn't sense Jodie, the person, the young person. She just seemed to ... She felt her lips tighten as the thought hit her. She just looks like an empty space.

> Sandy is being deeply affected by Jodie. The part of Jodie that was engaging with Sandy has suddenly apparently vanished. The young person so full of her enthusiasm towards her two friends has disappeared too. Both felt so real, yet one seemed so full, the other so empty. Sandy is becoming irritated with one aspect of Jodie, and this is going to cut across her ability to feel warm acceptance towards her, an important part of building a therapeutic relationship.

Jodie wasn't really thinking much; she felt pretty blank. She found herself feeling like this more and more these days. Something would happen and she'd just switch out. Didn't understand why. Didn't seem to happen to her friends. But it was how it was. It was cool.

She scratched the back of her head. 'Think I'd better go. Don't have anything to say here.'

'Feel like going, huh?' Sandy paused, allowing her empathic reflection to be heard, then she added, 'Nothing you want to say.'

Sandy was aware that she had stressed the 'you' in her response. That hadn't been intentional; it came out like that. It felt like it was coming out of her irritation. She regretted it immediately. Dammit, she thought, that's not how I want to express myself, but it is how I feel.

> Is Sandy congruent? She speaks in a way that she senses has been affected by
> her irritation. She senses this irritation to be emerging out of the contact she
> has with Jodie. At what point does it become appropriate to voice what she is
> experiencing? They haven't had much time together, and Jodie is not com-
> municating much verbally at the moment. Sandy wants to give it her best
> shot to form a therapeutic relationship. She has sought to be empathic. She
> has sought to hold an attitude of positive regard although she is finding this
> a struggle. Dare she be authentic insofar as expressing what she is feeling, or
> will that be too much, too soon?

Jodie looks up and notices that Sandy has a vague look on her face, like she is lost
in thought. Jodie could feel herself smile. Yeah, she thought, caught you not
giving me any attention. She felt good about it, felt she'd got one over on her.
Sandy came out of her thoughts and was aware of Jodie smiling momentarily
before she changed and resumed her previous facial expression. Yes, Sandy
thought, you caught me, but I caught you too.
'Seems like we can both get lost in our thoughts, Jodie. I was aware of how I was
feeling, kind of distant from you, like you were out of reach. And then I felt
really irritated, you know what that can be like, and then I came out of it and
noticed you smiling. Caught me out, huh?'
'You're supposed to listen to me, to, I don't know, not get irritated.'
'I'm a human being, I have my own reactions, we all do.'
'Yeah, well, but what about me?' Jodie was feeling kind of pissed off but also spoil-
ing for a bit of a verbal fight.
'What about you?' The response came from Sandy's instincts more than anything
else, a kind of triggered response.
'Well, I mean, you don't seem to say much.'
'No, neither of us are saying very much.'
'But sitting here saying nothing is just a waste of time, I mean, what's the point.
Shit, this is fucking crazy, you know. I come here and all you do is just sit
there. Fuck's sake.' Jodie was moving into anger and it wasn't just about
Sandy. However, she wasn't aware of this. All she could think of was what a
fucking waste of fucking time it was. She had better things to do, yeah, better
things to do.
'Gets to you, huh, really feeling angry about it?'
'Yeah, I mean, I don't know what to say, do I? I mean, you just sit there and I don't
know what to say. Fuck it, I need some help, you know what I mean? I need
some help here, and all you do is just sit.'
'Help? What kind of help?'
Yes, thought Jodie, got you. Now I'll really draw you in. 'Just want some time, you
know, just want to sort my head out. Yeah, that's it, I need to sort my head out.'
'Mhmm, stuff in your head needs sorting.'
'Yeah, I mean, my mum's a pain, yeah, she doesn't like what I do, doesn't like
anything I do. But I'm not gonna let that stop me. I've got my own life to lead.

I'm gonna do what I want. I want to smoke dope, I'll smoke it. I want to fuck around, I'll fuck around, yeah?'

'Yeah.' Sandy felt Jodie was pushing her, testing her out again, to see how she'd respond. She checked out that she had heard Jodie correctly. 'Yeah, you wanna do what you wanna do, smoke dope, fuck around, yeah?'

'Yeah.' Jodie went quiet for a moment. 'Yeah, that's right, know what I mean? Yeah. OK.' She felt surprisingly shocked that Sandy had just gone with her, hadn't given her some speech on what she should and shouldn't do.

'OK. Yeah?'

'Yeah.'

'Right, so, what now? What's with you now?' Sandy wanted to try and keep a focus on the immediacy of the encounter.

'Fuck, I don't know. I just tell you I'm gonna smoke dope and fuck around and you just let me say it.'

Sandy heard an emphasis on the 'just'. She replied with the same emphasis, more of an empathic reflection than empathic understanding. 'Sounds like you didn't want me to just let you say it.'

Jodie thought for a moment. 'Well, no, I mean, shit, I don't know what I want.'

Sandy sensed the confusion in Jodie's voice.

'Kind of confusing, yeah, kind of confusing.'

'I mean my mum, she'd go ape-shit if I said that, but not you. Why?' Jodie really couldn't understand this woman, this adult, she wasn't doing what Jodie expected, what she secretly wanted.

'Maybe I haven't got an agenda like she has? Maybe I really want to listen to you, get to know you, and not try and change you.'

Jodie jolted her head back. 'Come on, you're there to change me.'

'That's what you think, that I'm here to somehow make you change, make you stop doing something you want to do?'

'Yeah.' Jodie shook her head, 'I really don't get this. You're not gonna try and make me change what I'm doing?'

'No. But I do want to get to know you, understand you a little more, and maybe you'll get to know and understand me a little more too.'

> Sandy gives an open and honest response to Jodie. No games, no techniques, just a straightforward statement of what she hopes to gain from meeting up with Jodie in the counselling sessions.
>
> The exchange between them has become quite sharp and focused. Sandy is not expressing empathic understanding, but she is engaging with Jodie. There is a clarifying process taking place. Whether it is helpful, only time will tell. Perhaps Sandy is empathising with Jodie's need for confrontation but also to resolve her confusion. It is important for Sandy to maintain an attitude of warm acceptance and genuineness throughout this process.

Jodie shook her head, but said nothing. She hadn't dropped her face though; she was continuing to look at Sandy.

'Still confused, yeah. Look, let's level here. Your mum wanted you to come here so we could persuade you to stop smoking the dope, yeah? You decided to come back today because it might help get your mum off your case. That's the reality as I understand it.'

Jodie nodded, totally taken aback by not only what Sandy was saying, but the way she was saying it. She suddenly seemed quite calm yet very, very clear. It was like everything had suddenly shifted in some way. She felt somehow more focused. Yeah, what Sandy was saying was right, that was how it was. But she seemed to be saying it and being quite accepting of it.

Sandy continued: 'So here we are, two people, trying to be honest with each other, if that's what we want. I know I want to be honest with you, because I can't think of any other way I want to be.'

Jodie was listening now. 'Yeah, that's easy to say, but, I mean, it sounds real enough, but do you really care?'

Sandy felt the atmosphere quieten and intensify. 'Yes, I do really care, Jodie.' Sandy kept a very steady eye contact as she spoke, and her tone of voice was clear and quite matter of fact. No sickly sweet tones – generally a good indicator of a lack of authenticity.

Jodie didn't know what hit her. She couldn't believe it. She was crying. She didn't know why, but as she had heard Sandy speak she just suddenly felt tears welling up in her eyes and this hot lump form in her throat. 'I'm sorry.'

> The temptation is often to say something like 'No need to feel sorry' or 'It's OK'. Neither are empathic to the client's experiencing. The client has said sorry because they do feel a need to say 'I'm sorry', and they are not OK so why say 'It's OK'? Sandy responds to the underlying feelings.

'Hard to feel that care, yeah?'

Jodie nodded, while she tried to brush away the tears from around her eyes. Sandy reached across and got her a tissue which she passed over to her.

'You really meant that, didn't you, I mean, you really, really meant that?'

'Yeah.' Sandy didn't add any more, she did not see any need. She wanted to allow Jodie to be with what she was feeling, how she had reacted to what she, Sandy, had just said.

'I-I don't know why I reacted like that.' Jodie did know, but she couldn't say.

'Mhmm, your reactions, the tears, what you felt, you don't know why.'

Jodie shook her head. But she was thinking about how no one had ever really said anything to her quite like that, and in that way. No one. Her mum. Her sister. Her dad. Not like that.

Sandy sensed that Jodie was thinking about something, but she didn't want to intervene and somehow push her into disclosing anything she didn't want to.

> The person-centred counsellor is going to trust the client to voice what she needs to express. The counsellor is there to listen, to create a facilitative environment by offering the attitudinal qualities of the person-centred approach to encourage the client to emerge more fully into the therapeutic relationship.

Sandy took a deep breath. 'Phew, heavy stuff, yeah?'

Jodie nodded. She heard herself speaking, which felt strange as she hadn't intended to speak. Her voice sounded strangely quiet. 'No one ever said they care about me like that. Nobody.' Tears were welling up again. She closed her eyes and as she opened them again she looked down at her knees.

'No one, ever . . .'

Jodie was shaking her head.

'. . . said they cared about you.'

Jodie could feel her heart pounding. She wasn't sure how long it had been happening, but it was very strong now. She took a deep breath and breathed out slowly. She felt a rush of tiredness overtake her and she felt her eyelids getting heavy. She stifled a large yawn.

'Tired?'

'Yeah, and a bit spaced out too, like I've been smoking, you know . . .'

'Yeah.'

Jodie yawned again. 'But I haven't.'

'I believe you.' Sandy was genuine in her response.

Jodie heard the genuineness in Sandy's voice. That felt good as well, being believed. Not being questioned. She was aware that she was feeling more relaxed somehow, as well, although her back was tight between her shoulder blades. Probably how she was sitting, she thought. She moved around in the chair. 'Can't you get better chairs?'

'Blaming the chair, yeah?' Sandy knew she was smiling as she said it, and she noticed it triggered a smile on Jodie's face as well.

'Mum's always telling me to sit up as well.'

Sandy thought to herself that she hadn't said that, but it had been what Jodie had heard, or was she trying to wind her up?

Sometimes the counsellor will want to clarify what they meant; sometimes the encounter has moved on and it would disrupt the flow. However, it has informed Sandy of how sensitive Jodie is to being told what to do, or anything that she can interpret as meaning that. Such sensitivity is indicative of 'conditions of worth'. In this case Jodie knows she should sit a certain way to get her mother's approval, but then reverses this as an act of rebellion and so becomes more likely not to do what she is being told is good for her.

Conditions of worth can leave people behaving in certain ways to get approval, but they can leave someone – and this can certainly be the case for young people seeking their own independent identity – doing the opposite to affirm their individuality.

'Makes sense, huh?'

'Yeah, I guess she does sometimes.' Deep down Jodie knew she loved her mum, but she didn't often get in touch with that feeling. Usually she was too busy winding her up, reacting to her, ongoing battle, or so it seemed.

'Yeah, maybe sometimes she does.' Sandy was struck by this being probably the first positive thing that Jodie had said about her mother. It felt important, a significant shift. Jodie had connected with a fresh perspective, and seemed to have owned it.

'She must really hate me sometimes, you know?'

Sandy was aware of an instinctive frown as she replied in a questioning tone, 'Really hate you?'

'Yeah, I mean, I do give her grief.' She yawned again, and it triggered Sandy off as well. Sandy apologised. 'Sorry about that, they do seem to be catching.'

'It's OK, I started it.' She paused. 'You know, sometimes I just get so tired of it all.'

Humour can sometimes lighten things momentarily and allow the client to connect with and express something that they might otherwise have concealed. The person-centred counsellor does not apply this as a technique, but it can arise spontaneously and, as in this case, the comment about yawns being catching has perhaps allowed Jodie to disclose something she is tired of.

'Mhmm.' Sandy didn't say more, hoping to allow Jodie the freedom to continue as she felt she wanted to.

'Tired of all the battles at home, over what I wear, where I'm going, when I'll get back, my mobile phone bill, state of my room. Just wears me down sometimes, and that's when I smoke, you know, just to get away from it, to unwind, to just chill out. It's such a relief. Such a relief.' As she spoke Jodie could almost feel herself sinking into those wonderful, relaxing sensations.

'Sounds like you are halfway there now – such a relief from it all.'

Jodie nodded. 'Yeah. I like that feeling, and I don't want to lose it.'

'Yeah, it's important to you. You like to feel relaxed, you like to unwind, chill out. You don't want to lose it.'

'Talking about it now, I just feel so limp. And so tired still.' She glanced at the clock. 'How much longer have we got?'

'How much longer do you want? We finish at ten to at the latest.'

'I don't think I want to stay that long, want to give myself a bit of time before I meet up with Em and Ally. I want to be with them, but I want a bit of time to myself. Is that OK?'

'Sure. How are you feeling then now, other than tired?'

'Calm. It feels good. I don't feel so wound up.'

'Good feeling.'

'Yeah.' Jodie was nodding. 'Yeah, it is, and I got it without having to smoke anything!'

Sandy nodded and smiled.

There is no need for the counsellor to say any more. The client has made a clear recognition for herself. Better to let the client leave carrying her own words in her head affirming what she has realised, rather than the counsellors telling her what she has discovered.

The client is now trusted to use her insight however she needs to. The person-centred counsellor is unlikely to push any particular meaning, but allows the client to attach her own meaning to her experience.

They agreed to meet again the following week; however, the week after Jodie would be on holiday – a week in Cornwall with her parents and her sister.

Jodie left and spent a few moments sitting outside before she went to the bus stop. She felt good, calm, somehow less antagonistic towards Sandy. Something had changed during that session, and she was glad that it had. Maybe there was something to this counselling after all. She realised that she was very thoughtful as she walked down the road to get the bus. She was so lost in thought that she nearly didn't see them until they were right in front of her. Em and Ally. 'We thought we'd come and find you; didn't you get our texts?'

'No, no, I didn't. Guess I must have turned it off. Sorry.'

'You sound different. You OK, Jode?' Ally looked somewhat quizzically at Jodie.

'Yeah, yeah. Just feeling a bit odd, but yeah, I'm OK.'

'Counselling, huh, weird stuff,' Em commented, pulling a face.

'Yeah, it is, but it's good as well, Em.'

'Come on, let's go hit the town, go and see who's about.'

'And who we fancy most.'

They headed off, laughing, towards the bus stop, and Jodie forgot about the counselling. Yeah, time for some laughs with her best friends.

As for Sandy, she was feeling really pleased that what had felt such a difficult session had really developed in a way she had not expected, although she had learned long ago that in counselling you always expect the unexpected. She was particularly pleased that she had really caught some key moments that seemed to have helped Jodie shift in herself. It had felt really difficult, and then all that irritation inside herself, and then everything moved on. But it felt like they had engaged more, and particularly when she had heard herself say she was going to level with Jodie. Had she been irritated in that moment? It had felt quite powerful. And then the bit about caring. That really had affected Jodie, and maybe that had been too forcing, but it was said and done now.

She smiled as she thought about how she could justify herself – 'I was empathising with Jodie's combative nature, relating to her in a style she could relate to.' Maybe. Something had happened. It had been forceful. She could feel herself looking forward to the next session.

Points for discussion

- Reflect on the therapeutic impact on Jodie of Sandy's authenticity in the session.
- How do you deal with feelings that arise in sessions and which threaten to affect the accuracy of your empathy?
- What led up to and enabled Jodie to gain a shift of perspective towards her mother? How was this facilitated by Sandy?
- What are your thoughts on how forceful Sandy was, and the exchange over getting real?
- How would you have responded to Jodie saying the things that she was going to do? What reactions would you experience hearing this? What would you do with your reactions?
- If, before the session, Jodie had planned to smoke cannabis with her friends afterwards, do you think she will still do this? What factors will influence her decision?
- Write your own notes for the session.

CHAPTER 3

Counselling session 3: effects of the dope and a difficult dilemma

Jodie had begun talking about how it had been a shit weekend for her. She'd gone out to the cinema on Saturday afternoon and a party that evening. She talked a lot about the film, some comedy that seemed to be about a group of girls and how they had spent their time trying to attract the attention of some boys, but how it always seemed to go wrong. How there was one scene in some kind of coffee shop, or something, no, more of a café, and one of the boys was messing around with a ketchup bottle. Must have been blocked or something, and he was squeezing it to release it, and then it suddenly released and ketchup shot up and landed on his mate's head, and they'd ended up squirting it at each other before getting thrown out.

'And then they all went out, they hadn't eaten anything, and they walk into the burger place, you know, and they're covered in it and everyone just turns and stares, and it's just so crazy, you know? And they order their burgers and the guy serving them just doesn't say anything, he just stares. And this guy calls out, "Extra ketchup?", then he looks up, sees them and says, "Looks like you've already got yours", and starts laughing, and the whole serving area just goes hysterical. It's sooo funny. I nearly wet myself. They just stand there, the expressions on their faces, well, what you could see of their faces behind the ketchup.' Jodie was giggling as she described it and Sandy was left smiling too.

'The expressions, yeah, really got to you?'

'And then some other guy takes the bun off his burger, he's sitting near them, and just calmly reaches over with it and rubs it down the side of one of their faces, claps the burger back together and takes a big bite out of it. Nothing is said, they just turn and walk out, and the whole restaurant, everyone, just collapses in laughter.'

Sandy could just imagine it, some character just calmly reaching over to get his ketchup off the lad's face. 'Crazy stuff, huh?'

'Yeah. So that was really great.' Jodie described how they'd gone on to a burger bar themselves afterwards but couldn't stop laughing, and had to leave before they got to order their burgers. They ended up having pizza instead.

'Then we went on to this party. Someone's house from school. Birthday party.' She described what it was like, how they'd shared a joint, and there'd been a sleepover. She hadn't slept much. Felt awful all Sunday. 'Really weird. Don't know why. I mean, I just felt so uptight. I mean, dope's s'posed to chill you out, yeah, but I just felt really, really weird. Em and Ally were fine, didn't seem to affect them, but I really didn't like it.'

'So you think the dope affected you badly, got a bad reaction to it?'

Sandy thought she remembered Jodie saying something about not always feeling good with it before, but she wasn't sure. Anyway, she wasn't going to introduce that; she wanted to stay with her, help her explore what was happening for her. But she also wanted to check out how much Jodie was using; she had no clear idea. She held the question for a moment.

Jodie nodded. 'Yeah. Didn't like it. Did some more on the Sunday though, didn't want to say no. Would have felt, I dunno, kinda got a reputation to keep, you know? Don't want to look like I'm going soft.'

'That sounds really important to you, not to appear soft.'

'Yeah, I mean, it's all about respect, isn't it? I mean, I need respect from people. And I get it. Yeah, we do get a lot of respect.'

'Mhmm.' Sandy noted her curiosity as to who they got their respect from. But she knew that was her own personal curiosity and not a question with any therapeutic motivation. And besides, as a person-centred counsellor her primary role was to stay with the client, to be responsive to their frame of reference. 'Respect's what it's all about, yeah?'

'Yeah.' Jodie thought about how they got their respect, pressuring and taunting the younger kids. She didn't say anything about that though. Wasn't going to trust an adult with that.

'Jodie, I'm aware that I haven't a clue how much dope you're smoking, and I'm asking because, well, people can get really bad if they use a lot.'

'We share it, Ally and Em and me, we get it from Ally's brother. He seems to have enough. We don't get through a lot, about an eighth a week I guess, sometimes more. We had more at the weekend; there was a lot about at the party.'

Sandy thought about this and realised that it wasn't enough to be likely to trigger a psychotic reaction, not unless Jodie already had a predisposition towards this. Maybe she was just sensitive to it and it simply didn't agree with her. Or maybe she didn't always like the sensations she got. Or she was actually using more than she was saying.

'Only dope?'

'Yeah, well, and ciggies, and some booze. I guess I drank a bit too. But that's what you do at parties.'

'OK, so dope, ciggies and booze, yeah, and you were left feeling weird the next day.'

'Yeah, but the dope really makes the music good, I mean, you really get into it, seems to kinda sharpen it all up, really great. Yeah, the Saturday night was good, but the Sunday wasn't so good.'

'I guess I really want to try and help make sense of what it is that happens that gives you a bad reaction, Jodie. Did you smoke more?'

Jodie thought about it. It was a bit hazy. She could remember them getting up late that morning and heading off together. Somehow they'd wound up with a spliff each, yeah, that's right, not sure how or where they'd come from. Yeah, she'd smoked a whole one, and that was unusual, usually they shared, and usually what they shared wasn't so big either. 'I think I probably smoked a lot more than usual. Maybe that's what it was.'

'Mhmm. So what did it feel like? You say you felt weird, and I'm wondering what you mean.'

'Everything seemed sharper, sort of brighter. But that was only after I'd got really anxious. I don't know how long, but I felt really restless and then everything kind of settled down.'

'So, anxious and restless, and then calm, yeah, and things seemed brighter, sharper, clearer?'

'Yeah, and things seemed to look funny, well, yeah, just everything just seemed kind of stupid somehow. And that was OK, I was OK with that. But then I kind of felt like I was watching myself, I mean, that really was weird. Like I was kind of watching myself having these weird thoughts and feelings, never had that before. Started thinking everyone could see into my head. Didn't like that. But it passed and I kind of drifted back into a calmer state.'

'Quite a set of experiences, but it was the bit about watching yourself that really troubled you?'

'Yeah, and feeling people could see inside my head, like . . .' She shivered. 'That was bad.'

'You're getting kind of typical reactions to cannabis use, Jodie, and maybe because you had a lot more than usual you experienced them more strongly, or a more intense range than you have had before.'

'It was like I could see myself thinking and feeling, like I was watching, and then I kind of felt everyone could see me as well. Shit, I was really glad when it calmed down again.'

'Uhuh. Felt glad when the scary stuff ended.'

Jodie nodded. She really had been shocked by her experience and she really wasn't sure what she wanted to do about it. She hadn't said anything to Ally and Em, they seemed fine, but she knew she wasn't. But she didn't know what to do.

Sandy has checked out the cannabis use and the effects. This may not seem within a counsellor's remit, but given that Sandy has some knowledge and is experiencing genuine and realistic concerns, it seems an expression of unconditional positive regard to express that concern and to clarify what is happening, in case Jodie needs specialist assessment.

'I don't need to stop smoking dope, do I? I mean, I can't, I'd just well lose everyone's respect if I stopped.'

'It does sound like you are sensitive to it, Jodie, and the more you smoke, well, you may get to tolerate it more, but you may get more problems with it. It's not the harmless drug that some make out, you know. But I also want to respect your own choices on this as well. But I wouldn't be honest with you if I didn't say that I was concerned. It seems like a little shared out between you is OK, but more than that and you're in another world.'

'Yeah, and I don't like it, but I can't not use it. I can't.' She looked at Sandy, her eyes pleading for an answer. She looked so distraught, so sad and worried about her dilemma. Sandy's heart went out to her. Fifteen. Your two best friends doing something and you are realising you maybe can't do what they do, that you've got to find a way of not joining in, of being different. Shit, that's tough at any age, but 15. Sandy could remember her own teenage years. She never smoked tobacco, just never got into it. Remembered coughing when she tried it the first time, and just didn't persevere. Her parents hadn't smoked and she reckoned that may have helped. Now she was glad, but at the time, she just felt different.

'You can't not use it, but when you do you run the risk of feeling really bad, yeah. Tough one, that.'

Jodie was staring down again now, and picking at her nails. 'They're my mates, we share everything. I can't . . . I just can't . . .' Jodie was feeling really upset. She couldn't bear the thought of doing something that might affect her relationship with Ally and Em. She sat in silence for some minutes, still picking at her nails, and looking, well, the word that came to Sandy's mind was 'crumpled'. She'd lost her composure. She just looked totally deflated by her dilemma.

'Mhmm, you can't not use it, it's unthinkable to be different.'

Jodie couldn't get her head around it. They were mates. They did everything together. The words just kept going round and around in her head. We're mates; we do everything together. We do everything together. She shook her head and looked up at Sandy. 'I don't know what to do.'

'They're your mates; what do you do . . . ?'

Sandy has empathised with Jodie's dilemma; what does she do? This is not, however, a direct empathic response to her not knowing what to do. It has the effect of taking her from being with her not knowing to thinking about what she can do.

Jodie thought about it and wondered how they were going to react. They would believe her. Or would they? Might they understand? She couldn't imagine them taking her seriously, not at first. But she did need to say something to them and try and work something out. She wasn't sure that she was going to give up smoking dope, maybe the odd puff would be OK, maybe that would be OK.

'I need to talk to them, tell them how it is, you know. I don't know that I want to stop, but maybe I need to use it a lot less. I mean, it's not like I need it, it's just, well, it has been great. And part of me wants to carry on smoking and say fuck it, it's what I do, yeah? But I'm not sure about it any more.'

'Seems like you are really split, yeah, part of you wanting to carry on – fuck it – and another part is really not so sure about that.'

Sandy noticed the time; the session was heading towards a close, and she mentioned this but then brought the focus back to what she had just said in response to Jodie.

'Yeah, life's too short, yeah, I want to enjoy myself, have fun, have a few laughs, just do what I want to do.'

'What do you want to do, Jodie?'

Jodie went quiet. 'I want to have fun. I want to feel good. Fuck it. Yeah, I don't need this, it's doing my head in. I'm heading off.'

'OK, that's your choice, fuck it, have fun, feel good, does your head in thinking about it, yeah.'

Sandy knew that Jodie was going to head off and while she recognised that maybe this would be an opportunity lost, she also wanted to trust Jodie's own process. She maybe needed this reaction, needed to make her choices now and perhaps experiences would lead her to a different choice later on. She knew she couldn't make her do anything she didn't want to do, and that wasn't for her to do anyway. She had pointed out the risks and Jodie had heard that, but she was choosing to ignore it. She wanted to be with her mates, be like them, not be different. That was important to her, the most important thing, to belong, to be respected. Sandy respected that and she wanted to voice this before Jodie left. It felt like a critical moment. She wanted to be real.

'You want to be like Em and Ally, and yeah, that's really important. So good luck. I really mean that. As you say, life's too short. Enjoy!'

Jodie had started to get up, but sat down again. 'So you don't want to see me again?'

'I'd be really pleased to see you again, after your holiday – Cornwall, isn't it? But only if you want to come back.'

Jodie sat and thought about it. She really wasn't sure, but she felt she'd be most comfortable if she said yes. She didn't have to turn up. But it would avoid any lengthy discussion over it now. 'OK, same day, same time in two weeks, yeah?'

'Fine. See you then. Have a great holiday.'

'I'll try to, but it won't be easy. Still, I can keep in touch with Em and Ally. And it's only for a week.'

Jodie breezed out along the corridor, pleased to be heading off. It had left her feeling uncomfortable but she'd managed to push that aside. She was just going to do what she wanted; it was her life. She headed for the bus stop, pausing only to light up.

Sandy hoped she had conveyed to Jodie a sense of acceptance towards her thoughts and feelings towards the end of the session. She really wasn't sure. She knew she wanted Jodie to keep safe, but she didn't want to impose her concerns. She wanted Jodie to feel freed up to make her own choices, but she was concerned. She might be sensitive to cannabis, one of the people who did get bad reactions from it. Hell, some people went psychotic, could lose touch with reality. No one ever talks about that side of it much. But when you're 15 you have answers to everything. She hoped she would come back after the holiday. She kind of sensed that it was a bit in the balance. However, she wanted to trust Jodie's own process. She knew what she was experiencing and she needed to make her own choices. She would make the choice that best suited her, that gave her the greatest sense of satisfaction, that met her needs as she experienced them.

Points for discussion

- How concerned are you about Jodie's cannabis use?
- Would you have made different responses during the session and, if so, where and what might you have said?
- Do you think that Sandy's need for honesty, and the way she expressed herself towards the end of the session, was appropriate?
- Seeking to work to the principles of person-centred working can be challenging. Discuss the effectiveness and possible limitations of working in this way in this session.
- Will Jodie return for another session? Will she talk to Em and Ally? What might encourage her to do either or both from the session?
- Write your own notes for the session.

CHAPTER 4

Supervision 1: the counsellor explores her feelings and receives encouragement and support

'I've got a new client at the agency. Fifteen-year-old. Jodie. Referred in by her mother really; she'd found cannabis in her bedroom. Anyway, she didn't want to be there and made that pretty clear at the start, but the relationship has developed since then, although I'm not sure she'll come back after the last session.'

Courtney smiled. 'They don't often hang around, do they?'

'Well, it got uncomfortable for her and she's really caught between using cannabis with her friends, or not using or cutting back and risking losing her reputation and stuff.'

'Yeah, important stuff. So how does it feel being in relationship with her?'

A key feature of person-centred supervision lies in exploring the relationship that the supervisee has with their client and the feelings, thoughts and experiences that the supervisee has within that relationship. The emphasis is on helping them to reflect on their congruence, the quality and nature of their empathy and their ability to be warmly accepting of the client, and what may interfere with any of these – the intention being to clarify and to ensure that the supervisee is able to offer those aspects of the 'necessary and sufficient conditions' for which they have responsibility.

'It feels good and it feels challenging. I nearly said "felt", which I guess reflects my uncertainty as to whether she will come back.'

Courtney was nodding. 'Yes, that seems quite present.'

'I'm concerned and I guess I'm wondering whether I handled expressing that concern.'

'Can you say a little more?'

'Well, we got into exploring her cannabis use.' Sandy went on to describe the party and the effects the cannabis had had on Jodie the next day, and the dilemma she felt she was facing with her two best mates, Ally and Em, over it. As she spoke, Sandy could feel a sense of heaviness in her; it just felt so weighty to talk about. She voiced this.

'OK, so as you talk about this dilemma you can feel a real weight. In you, on you, around you?'

'Inside me, here.' Sandy put her hand over her tummy, just below the solar plexus. 'Feels kind of bulky as well.'

'So, weighty, bulky, in this area.'

As Sandy focused on it she realised that it was changing, dissipating and becoming more of an all-over sensation, but more on the edges of her body. 'It's shifted. It's more a kind of weight, no, more a kind of pressure all over my skin but it doesn't feel like it touches my skin. Makes me feel quite lethargic.'

'Lethargic, sort of not feeling motivated?' Courtney wasn't sure about that as he said it; somehow it sounded like he was trying to hang his own meaning on what Sandy was trying to say.

'No, she's motivated, but . . . I've switched to talking about Jodie, that's interesting. Wonder why I did that?'

'I wonder too.'

Sandy sat with her experiencing. She couldn't figure out why, but she had a clear image of Jodie sitting like she had for a lot of the sessions, sort of slumped in the chair, and picking at her nails. She described this to Courtney.

'That how you feel?'

'Yes, I guess it is, and I'm aware I feel quite tense as well, up here, in my shoulders.' She took a deep breath. 'Feels like I'm carrying something, something heavy.'

'Mhmm, I'm just wondering whether it was something you picked up when you were with Jodie.'

Sandy could still see Jodie sitting there, and the struggle she had had, saying how she couldn't change, that she shared everything with her mates. She thought about how the session had continued. How Jodie had switched into wanting to go, to get on and live her life. Shit, Sandy thought, she kind of left it behind, dumped the heaviness of it all on me, or at least I picked it up. Or did she just leave me more sensitive to my own stuff? 'You know, I don't know that I picked it up, but maybe she put me in touch with something in me. I don't know that I believe we pick up our clients' stuff unless we have something that kind of resonates to it within ourselves. I'm wondering what it may be in me that kind of got triggered by her dilemma, the weightiness of her struggle to decide what to do.'

'OK, so the question is what in you might in some way be similar to what Jodie was experiencing in that session?'

Sandy felt an overwhelming urge to stretch, which she did, and it felt good. Her back had become really tight and it felt energising to just open her arms out and move her back muscles.

'That looked satisfying.' Courtney smiled.

'Yeah, felt like I needed to expand a bit.' She paused to think for a moment. She thought about herself at Jodie's age. 'I never got out and about like she does when I was her age. Seemed to be at home most of the time. We lived in a fairly remote area. Didn't get out to many parties, but had the occasional sleep-over. Don't remember any drugs being around much though, just didn't really figure. Why did I stretch when you said about what might be similar in me to Jodie? She just seems so different, headstrong, out and about. Me, I was quiet, never really defied anyone. She just seems such a contrast.'

Courtney nodded and was struck by the difference. He wanted to ensure that Sandy knew he had heard this. 'I'm really struck by the difference between you, a real contrast.'

'Yes.' Then a powerful thought struck her, and it was powerful. One of those thoughts that she kind of knew, but then suddenly you really know it, like it becomes very immediate.

Courtney noticed Sandy's expression change. She had suddenly frowned. 'Yes?' he asked.

'Part of me would have so liked to have been like her, but would have been scared to death at the idea as well.'

'She kind of reminds you of how part of you wanted to be, but that also scared you as well.'

Sandy nodded. She could see some of the girls from her school; they just seemed so carefree, so liberated, she couldn't think of a better word, just seemed to have a 'not-care' attitude to life. She had always been so serious, and a little bit timid.

'I'm just thinking about some of the other girls at school and how they just seemed so cool, so . . . the word I had was "liberated", kind of freed up and con-fident. I was never like that, not really until I got into counselling. The training and the therapy changed all that.'

'But there is something about Jodie that kind of echoes from your past, of looking up to the other girls and wishing you were like them.'

'You know, I'm beginning to wonder if being with Jodie has kind of burst a bubble for me.'

Courtney frowned, unsure what Sandy was meaning.

'It's like maybe I've been carrying a secret desire to be like those girls – like Jodie is, at least – part of me has been carrying that dream, hope, call it what you will. And now Jodie has kind of burst it, shattered the dream. Made me – well, that part of me – realise that maybe it isn't as glamorous as I thought it was. Yes, the more I think about this, the more real it feels. Part of me I have carried, unno-ticed, and it has taken Jodie to come into my life to draw my attention to it.'

'She's given you quite a gift.'

'Well, I've often thought about how two-way this counselling is, how both the counsellor and the client learn through the process.'

> It does seem that counselling is a two-way process, that while the counsellor is offering an opportunity to their client, the client is generally offering something back to the counsellor as well. It can be helpful in supervision to reflect on what 'gift' the client has given the supervisor in terms of their experience of being with that client.

'Mhmm. So Jodie represents a dream that you have carried, kind of unwittingly, and suddenly the dream is seen through, no longer so glamorous.'

'No. And it seems to have left me more acutely aware of the risks that Jodie is taking, and I kind of feel that really did affect the way I was with her. I think I was maybe more concerned than I was aware of. I mean, she's not going psychotic on the cannabis, she's not smoking that much, but she didn't feel good after that spliff she smoked and maybe if she carries on, and maybe they smoke more, well, I guess I'm concerned. I know I'm concerned. Shit, there's part of me that wants to say, "For fuck's sake, Jodie, stop before it gets to you".'

'But you didn't say it?'

'No, and I don't know how much of that I was consciously aware of at the time, but I can certainly feel it now, and I'm left wondering if I'll see her again and whether an opportunity to make a difference in her life has been lost. And I really feel that.'

'Heavy feeling, huh?'

'Shit, yeah, that's what it is. Yeah.' In that moment it felt like something had shifted and lightened inside herself. There was something about being able to acknowledge it, but she was also aware of feeling angry with herself as well, and aware that she wanted to trust Jodie, to trust her own process. But the truth was, she knew she didn't, at least she didn't trust it to keep Jodie safe. And that was what she was feeling more than anything else. While she didn't have children herself, she felt that she wouldn't be letting Jodie do what she did without saying anything. Oh-oh. 'I think I have the capacity to be too much like Jodie's mother.'

'You look shocked.' Courtney responded to Sandy's facial expression.

'Well, I began wanting to form a relationship with Jodie. I didn't know anything and just felt that here was another young person who wasn't understood and was being taken to us to be "sorted out" and "told what to do". Which we don't do. But now, I think I have a lot more sympathy for the mother. Well, I mean, I seem to have feelings for both Jodie and her mother now, and I can just see the fix they are in. Her mum must be exasperated, and Jodie is just, well, potentially heading for problems if she is particularly sensitive to cannabis, or it leads to other, harder drugs. Not that it started with the cannabis; she's already smoking tobacco and drinking alcohol, so she was already on to the conveyor belt of mood-altering substances.'

'There seems to be a kind of inevitability in your voice, and I'm unclear where that's coming from. Not everyone does develop huge hard-drug problems from this kind of origin, though we know that many do.'

Sandy thought about it. She remembered something. 'Drugs are too close, too available. They get the cannabis from the brother of one of her friends, Ally I think, but I'm not sure. And that sense that they do everything together. I feel concerned that Jodie might have more problems with the substances. And I may be wrong, but it's what I sense, what I feel.'

'And it's important to acknowledge that, and I want to say that I really feel for you sitting with all these feelings, and I want to ask what you want from me to be able to, I don't know, manage, process – what's the right word? – *be* with what is present for you.'

> Encouraging the supervisee to reflect on their supervisory needs is important. The person-centred supervisor will want to be open to what their supervisee feels they need, and seek to offer this where possible.

'I think having the space to just be with all of this, but in awareness, not having it on the edge and sort of unknown to me, is hugely important. I feel I'm kind of owning myself, my reactions, and that feels important. Like I don't want to go back to being with Jodie with a load of stuff on the edge of my awareness that impacts on our relationship and I'm not conscious of the process. I want to be congruent, authentic. I want to know myself accurately when I am in the room with her, you know? I don't want stuff going off inside me that disrupts my congruence or distorts my ability to accurately hear what she is saying and communicate what I have heard. I want to ensure that I can be warmly accepting of her and not let some reaction in me to her behaviour get in the way of that. Yeah, I don't mind not feeling good about what someone is doing, but I still hope to feel warm towards them, as the unique person that they are.'

Sandy could feel herself becoming more passionate as she was speaking. She cared; she really did care about her clients. She wanted to be authentically present for them, and for herself. She knew she felt more satisfied in her own experience of herself when she felt she was being authentic. She believed in those necessary and sufficient conditions; she knew from experience that they challenged the client, and the therapist, in so many ways, and they provided a climate of relationship within which constructive personality change could occur.

Courtney felt wonderful listening to Sandy connect with her passion and her belief in the approach. She just seemed to come alive, such a contrast again to how she had been a few minutes before, struggling with the heaviness of it all. He really wanted to support her in this, acknowledge her strength of feeling. He knew he could say something jokey, but he also knew that would take away from the seriousness of the moment. Sandy was serious about her commitment to this way of working and he wanted to acknowledge the strength of that, support it, nourish it, encourage it. 'I'm really touched hearing you speak like that, puts me in touch with my own passion, but I want to honour yours. I want to say that Jodie has been lucky to meet you and I'm sure that you have affected her, even though she may not be aware of it. She's struggling with some really huge issues, particularly her street cred and being part of things with her mates. Hugely important stuff. You've listened to her, genuinely, and you've cared about her. Part of her may react against it, but other parts will recognise it like the seedling recognises which direction the sun is in.'

Sandy felt her eyes watering, particularly as she could see water in Courtney's eyes too. She swallowed. 'Thanks for that. Thanks. That image of the seedling, yes.' She blew out a deep breath, and she remembered something else from the sessions. 'I told her that I cared, I think it was in the second session. I forget how it came about, but it had a dramatic effect. It was one of those electric moments, and Jodie cried. She really heard and felt that care, I think. It really affected her. She said no one had ever expressed caring for her quite like that. It seemed to calm her, and she even said she felt more understanding towards her mother, acknowledged how much of a pain she must be.'

'Powerful, powerful stuff. You really connected with her.'

'Yes, but now she's disconnected.'

'From?'

'Me.'

Courtney could sense Sandy blaming herself, though she hadn't said it; it was the way she bit her lip after her response. 'Whose problem is that? Maybe she needs to . . . for now. Part of her may feel threatened by the powerful experience she had with you. But she has felt your care, part of you has felt that, and that part won't forget it.'

Sandy nodded. 'Sown a seed, I guess.'

'And it will want to look for the sun.'

Sandy smiled. 'Yeah, but there are some chemicals around that may destroy that seed, Courtney, it may not get a chance to germinate, that's what worries me.'

Courtney nodded. 'Yeah, and there is no answer to that one. That's the tough realisation we all have to face, particularly working with people starting out using substances. How will they grow and develop, how much can they realise their potential as people, and what part will the substances play in that, either negative or positive?'

'Yeah, I know, so much creativity in our world has been drug-induced – how many classical composers used substances to heighten their experiencing to pour into their music, and not just classical, of course.'

'And poetry, and art, and all kinds of creativity.'

'But I also see the damage as well, the fallout, the wasted opportunities, and with new substances being designed, we don't have a clue what the long-term effects are.'

'And so many young people don't live in a long time-frame. Those that do may have greatest resilience, but those who are into the experience of the moment – and that may be because what they see ahead is bleak and unacceptable, or it may simply be they want to feel good now and have found a fast way to achieve it chemically – they're not in touch with the idea of potential or actual long-term effects.'

Sandy nodded. 'I can feel quite depressed by it all at times.'

'You work in a tough environment, emotionally demanding. You care and you are effective because you care, but you are also affected because you care. But that care reached out and touched Jodie, and she won't forget that. It's gone in deep.'

'I need to hang on to that. Thanks for reminding me. I just wish I knew what was going to happen next, but then, maybe I don't. I just hope she turns up for the next appointment.'

'Yeah, you really do want that. I hope so too, and if she doesn't, well, maybe she has a good reason and she will get back in touch for more of that sunlight.'

Points for discussion

- How would you sum up the content of the supervision session? Were the issues covered that in your view needed to be covered?
- Evaluate Courtney's responses to Sandy. Was he staying with a person-centred philosophy of working?
- After reading through the supervision session, are you left feeling differently about Jodie, Sandy, young people, drug use? And if so, what is that difference?
- Reflect on the importance of the supportive element as a feature of supervision.

CHAPTER 5

Counselling session 4: Jodie doesn't attend

It was ten minutes after the time that Jodie was due. There had been no word from her and Sandy was aware of feeling anxious. The session with Courtney had helped her to feel a lot clearer in herself, and she really wanted to be there for Jodie if she wanted to come back and re-engage in the therapeutic relationship.

The minutes continued to tick by as she sat, reflecting back over the previous sessions. Whatever Jodie chooses, she has her reasons to make that choice. She was concerned still that what could start out as free choices, particularly around drugs, could soon become a drive, a need, and eventually an addiction. But she also didn't want to overreact. There was a softer, caring part of Jodie; she had seen it emerge in that second session. Perhaps it didn't often get a chance to appear.

More time had passed. It looked like Jodie wasn't going to come. She was sorry and decided to spend a little while being with her reactions to the situation. How did she feel? What was present for her? Yes, there was anxiety. She pondered on the many reasons why Jodie might not have arrived, and she realised how much she had been making huge assumptions – there were so many reasons. It didn't necessarily mean she didn't want to come; perhaps something else that seemed more important had come up. The truth was she didn't know, and she realised it was pointless sitting and speculating. She needed to offer her another appointment. Oh, she thought, now what's the best way of doing that. I want it to be confidential. Would her mother respect a letter's confidentiality? She hadn't checked with her in that first session. She should have done. Damn, she thought. She had her mobile number though. She was loath to phone; she always felt that was invasive. Clients might be making a genuine choice not to come and that needed to be respected. Chasing them down wasn't going to be therapeutically helpful. Sometimes it was a valuable experience for a client to not come and to find that they weren't going to get criticised, but rather offered an opportunity to understand why.

She decided to text her, just a brief message to say she hoped she was OK, that she was sorry she hadn't made it, and that she could see her next week at the same time. She felt that was the best course of action to take. But she decided to leave it until later, until after the session would have finished.

Counselling session 5: the relationship develops, giving Jodie tough choices

Ten minutes into the session again and still no sign of her. Sandy was beginning to feel resigned to the fact that, for whatever reason, Jodie was not going to arrive. She decided to make herself a drink and was just heading off to the kitchen when the receptionist called her. Jodie had arrived. Sandy went out to find her.

'Hi. Come on through.'

Jodie walked along the corridor silently and entered the counselling room, plonking herself down once again in her usual position.

'So, it's good to see you. I realise you didn't make it last time, but you're here this week. How do you want to use the time?'

Sandy deliberately did not ask about the no-show the previous week. She would leave it for Jodie to mention this if she wanted to. She was mindful of wanting to check about contacting her in the future. Obviously the text message had got through, but she knew she needed to clarify this.

'Yeah, sorry about last week, but mum was on my case so much, I just got fed up with her telling me what to do and what was good for me, you know? So I didn't come. Went to the cinema instead. Of course, hadn't turned my mobile off, had I? Your message bleeped and I had to rummage around for it.'

'Good timing, or bad timing?'

'You know that bit where they have that bit from *Jaws* and he's looking around and they play the mobile phones to make you turn yours off. Well about ten seconds after that was when mine bleeped!' Jodie was smiling about it. They'd all giggled at the time and got told to 'sshhhh' by the people behind, which actually just made them giggle even more.

'So more bad than good timing, though I'm glad it entertained you all!'

'It kind of made me realise that I maybe should have been here, but it also felt good not coming as well. Like, it felt like I needed to make my own decision, do what I wanted, not what my mother wanted.'

'She wanted you to come?'

'Yeah. Didn't tell her I'd bunked off though.'

'Feels good, doesn't it, bunking off, doing what you want to do?'

Sandy empathises with the feelings. She preserves a non-judgemental attitude, wanting to offer Jodie the opportunity to explore rather than sound critical, which could leave her defensive and less open to her own experience and to sharing it.

Jodie nodded, quite vigorously, and smiled. 'You're not going to tell me off about it, are you?'

'No. You expected me to?'

'Sort of, I mean, people do, don't they? But I wasn't sure. You've been different and that kind of confuses me. I mean, some of the things you've said haven't been what I expected, but they've felt good, but it's confusing.'

'So your usual experience is to get told off, yeah, when you don't do something that someone else expects of you. And the way I am with you is confusing.'

'Yeah. It's like you can't ever do what you want without someone saying no.'

'You don't like people stopping you doing what you want to do?'

'I don't. I mean, it's parents usually, and teachers. They're sometimes worse. Always think they know best.'

'You don't like that.'

'They don't always know best and they won't listen. They just tell you to do what they say, but don't give you a reason or nothing, just tell you what to do, and what not to do. I just want to do what I want.'

'It's hard, isn't it, when people tell you what they think is good for you and it's different to what you think.'

> Sandy has missed the 'I just want to do what I want' and has unwittingly directed her away from this aspect of what she has just been experiencing.

'Don't like it. But you're different and that's why I'm confused. I talk about our sessions to Em and Ally and they think it's really cool. In fact, they both talked of coming along, see who this weird woman is who kind of listens and tells you that she cares and doesn't tell you what to do. And that made me feel really good, like I had something special, and yet I didn't want to share it. And that's different. I mean, you know, we share everything. But not this. Somehow this is mine, and I don't know why, but I want this for myself. And then I go to the cinema, but that wasn't about this, that was 'cos of my mother going on at me.'

'So Em and Ally want to come, but you want to keep this special for you, but you end up going to the cinema as a reaction to your mother? I can appreciate that, Jodie.'

Jodie pulled a face.

'What did I say?'

'Well, do you have to call me Jodie? It's what my parents call me and, well, they're usually being critical or something and, well, my friends call me Jode and I feel more comfortable with that.'

'OK, so you want me to call you Jode?'

Jodie nodded.

'OK Jode, no problem. And I want to say I feel honoured; I really mean that. I think it kind of says something about I guess how you view me and the counselling.'

> Jodie is no longer seeing Sandy as the authority figure that she may have thought she was before. She is now being invited to address her, and therefore relate to her, more as a friend. The relationship is developing.

'Yeah. Yeah. I've never really talked to anyone like this before and it feels good.'

'Mhmm, feels good.' Sandy didn't voice her curiosity as to what felt good, realising this would have been directing her away from her here-and-now experience.

Jodie sat in silence. She really wasn't sure what to say now. She kind of felt like she ought to say something, but she wasn't sure what. Eventually she spoke. 'So, what now?'

'Anything in particular you want to talk about?'

Jodie thought about it. 'Don't know really. Not a lot has happened. Holiday was sort of OK, though, you know, a week with your parents,' she blew air through her teeth, 'not the highlight of the year. But at least I got a tan, and met this guy who was staying at the same hotel. Oh yeah, fancied him. Nothing happened though. Spoke to him a bit, watched him swimming and stuff. Got his mobile and we've texted a bit since then. Lives miles away. But that feels good.'

Sandy noticed a little extra colour in Jodie's cheeks as she was talking about him. 'You really liked him, yeah?'

'Yeah, I did, but I felt, I don't know, kind of didn't know what to say. I mean, that's not like me. When Em and Ally are with me, well, we'll chat up anything in trousers, well, almost, I mean, we do have some standards.' She smirked.

Sandy smiled and responded to the content of what Jodie had said. 'So you felt somehow, what, more awkward on your own trying to talk to this guy?'

'Yeah, felt all kind of funny inside. Em and Ally told me I was in love, and I told them I wasn't and pushed them away. They keep teasing me. I kind of like it but I don't as well, like I feel really kind of weird inside.'

Sandy could feel a kind of curiosity about this guy, and she wanted to know more, and she knew that was the 'sitting-in-a-café-catching-up-on-the-gossip' part of herself, not appropriate for counselling. 'Mhmm, their teasing leaves you feeling all kind of weird.'

'Yeah, and I keep thinking of him, you know? He'd got wonderful blue eyes, drop-dead gorgeous. And ...' She had coloured up again and suddenly felt all shy and self-conscious. She sort of put her hand across her forehead, trying to hide her embarrassment.

'Kind of gets to you, blue eyes, drop-dead gorgeous, can't get him out of your head.'

'No. I just keep thinking about him. I want to keep texting him, but I can't, I mean, not all the time. Mum already goes on at me about how much I use it. But I just can't wait to hear from him. He texts me and I reply straight away and then, oohh, I have to wait. Guess he's like me, can't send too many texts, probably got his parents on his case as well.'

'So you reply straight away and then have a long wait, and you can't wait to hear from him.'

'It's horrible and wonderful all at the same time. Does that make sense?'

'Does to me; how about you?'

Jodie nodded. Yes, she thought, that is how it feels. And it does feel good talking about him even though she had felt embarrassed. Now she had started it seemed a lot easier.

Sandy was aware that Jodie hadn't mentioned his name and she thought about asking.

Working with an adult the counsellor is probably going to be less likely to ask what his name is; however, with a young person there are often different boundaries. Young people have different agendas. They may see the counsellor less as a professional and more as a kind of friend, someone they can confide in. Jodie is clearly finding it easier to be with Sandy. The therapeutic relationship is being built. It is allowing her to explore herself more freely, and to experiment with how she is. It has become quite precious to her, not something she wants to share, even with Em and Ally.

Part of building a therapeutic relationship with a young person involves taking an interest in their lives and interests, but without coming across like 'The Spanish Inquisition' (Monty Python). Nobody expects etc. ... Sandy decides to enquire.

'So, what's his name then?'

'Desmond, though he likes to be called Des.' She'd coloured up again. 'Why can't I talk about him without this happening. And why have you got a silly grin on your face?'

'I'm sorry, Jode, I really am.' She was, but she couldn't get the smile off her face.

'I'll forgive you; at least you remembered my name!'

'Yeah, I do listen. So, Desmond, or Des. And it seems like he's taking up a lot of your time at the moment.'

'Yes.' She rubbed her nose. 'Yes, feels good.'

'OK, great, so . . .' Sandy glanced at the clock. About 15 minutes or so left.

Jodie noticed her glance.

'So, how do you want to use the rest of the time?'

Sandy does seem to mention the time quite a lot. It can, as perhaps in this case, be interpreted by the client as meaning, 'I've had enough listening to what you have been saying, what now?' This needs to be avoided, or the client should be offered the opportunity to continue with what they are currently exploring.

'I guess I want to talk more about what you were saying last time. Like, I know I said about wanting to do my own thing, live my own life and stuff, and I do, but, well, I guess I'm kind of unsure about the pot. I mean, I feel OK about it really, but I'm not sure. Haven't smoked much since I've been back from holiday. I mean, we've had some, but I haven't really smoked as much as I had in the past. Em and Ally don't seem to have noticed that much. I still get an effect, but I guess I'm kind of uncertain about it, you know?'

'Yeah, so you haven't smoked as much dope, still get, what, enough of an effect? And Em and Ally don't seem to have noticed?'

'No. And I haven't really talked to them about it. That was a part of our – what do you call this, contacts, conversations, whatever – anyway that was a part that I didn't talk to them about.'

'Hard to talk to them about it, yeah?'

'I don't think they'd take me seriously. Sometimes I begin to feel kind of different. At other times, I feel the same, you know, fooling about and stuff with them really like that. And then there are times when I kind of feel, I don't know, different.'

'So sometimes you feel like you always did, and at other times you feel different.'

Jodie nodded. 'Like I feel I'm kind of, oh I don't know, I was going to say changing. Like I want to be with them, but sometimes I don't. Like now. I actually want to be here talking like this. I don't want them to be part of this. But then when I hear myself say that I feel bad about it.'

'Like part of you wants to be with them, but now there's another part of you that wants different things, one of them being here?'

'Yeah, and that's kind of new, and I guess in a way it seems really linked to coming here.'

Sandy nodded.

It is likely that what is occurring is the development of a new configuration within Jodie's structure of self (Mearns, 1999; Mearns and Thorne, 2000), which is in direct response to the experience she is having of a person-centred relationship in the counselling sessions.

'So it's like a new part of you.'

'Yeah, and it feels good but it feels kind of not me.'

'Feels good but it doesn't feel like you.'

Jodie was shaking her head. It was very confusing for her. She really didn't know what to make of it. It didn't feel really scary, but it did feel kind of unsettling somehow, hard to describe; she just knew she was different.

'It's kind of serious.'

'It feels serious?'

'Yeah, like part of me wants to kind of think about things a bit more, not just rush in . . .' Jodie paused before continuing, speaking a little quicker. 'But I like rushing in too!'

'And the thought of rushing in makes you smile whereas the serious part leaves you, well, looking serious.'

Jodie sat quietly, for perhaps a minute, but she wasn't slumped in the chair any more. She seemed more alert, as if there was more going on in her head. Sandy voiced her perception. 'You look somehow more alert and thoughtful; you're even sitting differently.'

'I guess I am. But I'm not sure what to do.'

'Mhmm, not sure what to do.'

'I kind of want to just be me, but I'm not so sure who me is any more. It's kind of good to be thoughtful, you know, but I like goofing around with Em and Ally as well.'

'You make it sound like you can't have both.'

> This has come from Sandy's frame of reference, not Jodie's. Sandy is experiencing her as saying she can't have both, but she is not actually saying this. Jodie is simply stating that she likes both being on her own and being with Em and Ally.

Jodie stopped and thought about it. 'I suppose I can have both. I guess ...' She didn't have a chance to speak, her mobile bleeped – text message. Jodie clicked it up on to the screen. It was Ally wanting to know when she was going to be let out; they were at the bus station. As she had reached for the phone she'd really thought it would be Des, she really hoped it would be Des. She was disappointed that it was Ally.

'Ally, wanting to know when I'll be "let out". I'm not going to reply now, she can wait.'

Interesting, Sandy thought; the session is more important than Ally and Em, at least it is when Jodie is in the place in her self that she is at the moment. She held her on the experience with a question. 'Sure you don't want to reply?'

'No. Where was I?' She'd lost her train of thought.

'You were saying that maybe you could have time for the thoughtful you and time to goof around with Ally and Em, and you started saying something, "I guess ..." and then your mobile bleeped.'

Jodie thought about it, but it had gone. She felt irritated. That was unusual. She never felt irritated with either of them. 'I don't know, but I do feel irritated.'

'By ... ?'

'The text message. I'll turn it off next time. I'll turn it off now, they can wait a few minutes. It's nearly time to go.'

'You really are serious about this space, this time, being for you, aren't you?' Sandy was struck by the importance of this decision. Fifteen-year-old girls, their friends and their mobiles seemed inseparable. Jodie was changing, something was happening for her, and she felt a responsibility to be there for her through this process.

'I really regret not coming last week, but I don't want to blame them. I made the decision. I kind of need to go and think about all of this. But they're waiting for me and I really feel I need to see them. Like I can't do both.'

'Can't do both. What to do?'

'I don't want to go home, and I don't really want to be on my own, so maybe I'll go and meet up with them. I'm still confused.'

'Change can be confusing, but it seems that you have made a decision for this time.'

'Yeah.'

'OK, time's just about up. Same time next week?'

'Yeah, that's cool. I'll see you then.'

'OK.' Just as Jodie was getting up Sandy remembered about contacting her. 'Oh, I meant to ask, if for any reason you don't get to a session and I don't hear from you, is it OK to send a new appointment by text, or should I send a letter? I was concerned if I sent you a letter whether it would get opened by someone else?'

'No, they're good about that. I get my own post, though mum does hover around sometimes to see who it's from. I'd prefer a text. And I'll try not to be in the cinema next time!'

'OK. See you next week. Take care.'

'Yeah. Bye.'

Jodie headed off to find her two friends. Sandy followed her along the corridor and noticed that she hadn't got her mobile out. She's going to have a tough time, she thought, really pulled in different directions. And she, Sandy, was contributing to it. But she recognised that Jodie was choosing to engage with her, that clearly some aspect of her wanted this kind of experience.

From a person-centred perspective we can think of it as the actualising tendency having shifted focus into this newly forming configuration with the self. Rogers described this tendency as 'the directional trend which is evident in all organic and human life – the urge to expand, extend, develop, mature – the tendency to express and activate all the capacities of the organism, or the self' (1961, p. 351).

In this instance we might regard this 'urge to expand, extend, develop' to be finding a creative and expressive focus through this new focal point of experience. It therefore becomes the place within Jodie that develops a degree of primacy. Of course, this may not be maintained. Other configurations will seek to re-assert their control. It is likely to be a tough and confusing time for her, and only time will tell how she will develop through this process. She has a part of herself that has been constructed through the experience of the attitudinal values of the person-centred approach, and this will present a challenge within her structure of self that has developed in response to the more negative conditioning and introjects that perhaps had dominated her development in the past.

Points for discussion

• What do you think about the contrast between working with young people and adults? Do you think the counsellor needs to make adjustments?

- What other configurational parts do you think are present within Jodie, and how might they have developed or arisen?
- Was Sandy right to not mention Jodie being late for the session? Discuss the therapeutic value of raising this, and of not raising this.
- How important is the offering of warm acceptance to a client? What impact did it have on Jodie in this session?
- Write your own notes for this session.

CHAPTER 6

Counselling session 6: fear of becoming a woman

Jodie came into the counselling session, seemingly more purposeful given the manner in which she was walking.

'Shit, what a week.'

'Sounds difficult, or am I making an assumption?'

'No, difficult. I don't know, I'm finding I don't want to go out so much, just spending time at home, in my room. Just not so interested in stuff the same, and I don't know why. Haven't seen Em and Ally as much. Weather's been awful as well, hasn't really made me feel like going out either. Just can't be bothered.'

'So, you're in quite a lot then . . .' Sandy didn't complete her sentence.

'Yeah, kind of got into getting up later and listening to music and stuff. Just doing a lot of thinking, and I guess a lot of not-thinking as well. Just chilling out, and it feels OK. It feels good. Mum's around but not really pestering me much, probably glad I'm at home and not "wandering the streets" as she likes to put it. Dad's at work. My sister, yeah she comes in as well some of the time, but she's also out with her friends, or they're round at ours. She's a lot younger – ten, Karen. We kind of get on some of the time, but not that much. Anyway, so I've been in a lot and I guess what's been strange is that I haven't missed Em and Ally. We have met up a few times, and it's been good, I've enjoyed it, but somehow I like to come home as well. And that just isn't me, but now it is. Weird.'

Sandy was aware that Jodie had told her a lot and she wanted to check out that she had got it all clear.

> Often, empathic responses are in reality motivated from a desire by the counsellor to check out that they have heard and understood the client as the client intended. Empathy is not a simple technique of repeating back what the client has said.

'Can I just check out that I've got all that? You have seen Em and Ally a few times and enjoyed being with them, but you're also enjoying being at home and that's kind of different. Your sister is around some of the time, Karen, but she's often playing with her friends. And your mum hasn't been pestering you. But this idea of feeling good about coming home, that's weird.'

'How do you remember it all? I can't remember things. I go into shops to buy something and then can't remember why I went in. Crazy.'

'I want to remember; it's important for me to hear what you say so we can understand it.'

'Couldn't do your job. I'd want to tell everyone what to do, sort them out. They'd have to do it as well. Or else ...'

'Or else?'

'They'd be in deep shit!'

'Interesting style of counselling, might work for some people.'

'Well that's me, upfront, kind of what you see is what you get.'

'And what do they get, Jode?'

Another example of banter which is serving to strengthen the relationship. Yet, as we can see from what follows, Sandy has not lost sight of the therapeutic focus and it is close at hand.

'Well, they used to get someone who didn't give a damn what they thought about me, who just did what she needed to do to get what she wanted. Now, I'm not so sure.'

'So you're not sure that you are that person who didn't give a damn what they thought about you and did what you needed to do to get what you needed to get.'

'It's like, all too much effort. Like, what's the point. What is the point.'

'What's the point – seems more like a statement than a question.' Sandy could feel the atmosphere shifting in the room, getting heavier somehow. She instinctively felt she needed to be extremely focused.

'Well, I mean, what is there for me? I'm not doing too good at school, don't see myself going to college or university or anything, don't know what I want to do. Used to just think life was for laughs, but now, well, it's kind of serious. What the fuck am I gonna do with my life, huh?'

'Serious and big question, Jode, what are you going to do with your life?'

She shook her head. 'I don't know. I don't know what I want, but I know I'm changing but that seems to be making it worse. Makes me think about things more. I don't know, I don't seem to enjoy myself, at least, not this last week. Maybe it's the rain, I don't know, but it feels more than that. I mean, I feel OK staying at home, listening to CDs and stuff, and just chilling out, but when I think about it, think back over the day, I just feel kind of, I don't know, somehow dissatisfied. It feels OK at the time but when I think about it, it just seems like it's boring.'

'So, yeah, feels OK at the time but when you think about it later you feel like you're getting boring.'

> Sandy has not tried to reflect back all that has been said; rather she has reflected back the conclusion that Jodie has come to. This allows the flow to be maintained, yet Sandy has communicated that she is listening and in touch with what Jodie is communicating.

'Just feel like I'm not interested in things like I used to be, and it feels like it's all happening quite quickly. Des stopped texting me too, and I don't know why. And that was awful. He hasn't replied now for days. Em and Ally wanted me to send him a really rude message, but I couldn't. Didn't want to maybe upset him. I mean, there may be a good reason why he hasn't responded, I don't know. I just don't know. I feel so fucking miserable.'

Sandy was aware she was hesitating, unsure how to respond. She realised she was actually protecting Jodie from exacerbating her misery, but she wanted her to know she had heard what she said. She responded. 'Yeah, makes you fucking miserable, and you said it with a sigh.'

'How can I feel better? I don't like feeling like this. I don't know where I am, who I am, anything. I feel awful.' Jodie put her head in her hands and began to cry.

'Yeah, it's awful not knowing.'

Jodie sort of nodded although she still had her head in her hands and was continuing to cry. Eventually she took a tissue and dried her face. 'I don't feel good about myself at the moment, and I don't know what to do. What do I do?'

'You just so want an answer, Jode, about what's making you so miserable and what you can do about it. Just to get away from what you are feeling.'

Sandy's heart went out to her. She was really struggling, poor lass. Change could be so difficult, trying to come to terms with life, the present and the future.

Jodie was nodding again. Sandy took that as a response. She continued. 'What is it really, deep down, that's making you so miserable, Jodie?'

'I'm afraid, fucking terrified . . .' She stopped.

'About?' Sandy spoke softly, wanting to help Jodie say what she needed to say and not speak in such a way that it drew her attention away from her own experiencing.

'Life. The future. Being a woman. It's all so scary, and I can't cope with it all.'

'Life is scary, isn't it? The future. What will happen. And how it will be to be a woman.'

Jodie was nodding, still crying, but nodding through the tears. She took another tissue.

Sandy didn't say anything more; she sensed that the tears had begun to ease and she wanted to allow Jodie the space to come through the tears in her own way and at her own pace. Jodie sat for a while longer, sniffing, dabbing at her eyes. Finally she blew her nose, closed her eyes and took a deep breath. 'Oh God, I feel awful.'

Sandy had a real sense of loneliness, of how lonely it must be for Jodie. It didn't seem like this was something she could talk seriously about with Ally and Em, and Sandy didn't seem to be picking up that she was talking to her mother. 'I kind of sense that you haven't talked to anyone else about this.'

Jodie shook her head but said nothing.

'Not easy. Can feel so overwhelming and leave you feeling so alone with it.'

Jodie nodded her head. She had opened her eyes and was looking down at the floor to her right. She didn't know what to say. She just felt absolutely terrified and she couldn't do a thing about it. She felt terror and numbness at the same time. She felt totally stuck in the seat, yet wanting to run away from everything and everyone, and from herself. 'I'm so scared, Sandy, so scared.' Her voice had gone very quiet.

Terrified, awful, scared. Jodie has used all these words and Sandy has not responded empathically to any of them. Jodie may be left feeling not heard and not understood. Sandy has come back with loneliness, but this is not what Jodie has been saying. Sandy is oblivious to what is happening. Perhaps she felt similarly and has forgotten. We do not know. But it is an example of how empathic contact can be lost. The person-centred counsellor will be striving to avoid this occuring. But it can and does happen.

'Yeah.' They both lapsed into silence. Jodie felt unable to speak; Sandy didn't know what to say. She had no response. Jodie was facing a terror that was real to her and there was no denying its reality. Jodie was terrified of growing up. And Sandy immediately started thinking about how at risk Jodie might be, but pushed that aside. She wasn't going to introduce something and put some idea in her head that wasn't there because of her own anxieties.

The silence continued. It felt oppressive. It didn't feel healthy to Sandy. She was concerned as to how Jodie was feeling and what the silence was doing to her. 'I'm here if you want to say something.' Jodie sat, still staring, not moving. The thought went through Sandy's mind: can I trust her process here? Can I really trust her process, that what is happening inside her is necessary and will have a constructive outcome, eventually? She struggled with it. The thought of Jodie going home feeling like this left her very anxious.

Sandy sought to maintain her own congruence, maintaining an openness to her own experiencing. Yes, she was anxious and she allowed that to be present. She was concerned, and it was rooted in her clear recognition that Jodie was facing something that was enormous and potentially overwhelming, and which could lead to all kinds of problems: self-harm, eating disorders, even suicide. Yet at the same time she was not losing sight of her compassion for Jodie which was also very present and which she sought to hold in her awareness.

Jodie was feeling paralysed with fear of the future. She had this overwhelming sense of everything being out of her control. Her body was changing, her role in life would change, she would ... She couldn't imagine it. She couldn't see herself as a mother. She couldn't see it. But it was there, out there, waiting for her, waiting for her ... She felt herself taking a deep breath and as she breathed out her awareness shifted and she was aware again of Sandy. Well, she hadn't lost awareness of her, but now she was somehow more aware of her presence. She still felt unable to say anything. But she could move. She looked over to Sandy and met her eyes. As their eyes met she felt another shift, a sense that someone was there, someone cared, that she was alone but strangely not alone. She managed to speak, very quietly. 'I'm scared of what will happen in the future, my future.'

Sandy nodded, slowly and only slightly, tightening her lips before responding, 'Yeah, it's a real scary thing to think about, the future, your future.'

'No one else seems to see it like I do. Em and Ally just laugh about it all, they talk so easily about being mothers and wives and stuff. Me, I guess I'm different.'

'Different to them, yeah?'

Jodie nodded, and took a deep breath. 'Yeah. But it's gonna happen, and I have to face it, don't I?'

'It's going to happen, yeah, and you will face it.' Sandy was aware as she spoke that she was encouraging Jodie rather than being simply empathic.

Jodie went quiet, but this was a different quiet, more reflective. She was back in touch with her thoughts again, able to think about it all. 'I don't know if my mum will understand. I'd really like to try to talk to her, but I don't know if she will understand.'

'That's a real fear for you, Jode, will she understand, but you really want to try and talk to her.'

'Yeah, I have to. But it feels like an enormous step to take. I mean, we don't talk about things, you know, sort of serious things.' She smiled, but only slightly. 'It's usually her telling me what to do, and me not doing it!'

'Yeah.'

Jodie isn't really saying much about her feeling about growing up; she is choosing not to explore this at this time, and Sandy is not pushing her to. The person-centred counsellor stays with the client, allowing them to communicate what is present for them, trusting the flow of their experiencing to take them where they need to go, encouraged by the presence of the facilitative climate of relationship.

'Growing up ...' She shook her head and took another deep breath. 'But I'll get through it, Sandy, I have to, don't I?'

Sandy nodded. 'Yeah, you'll get through it.'

Jodie felt good talking to Sandy like this. She felt close to her. 'Wish you were my mum,' she said quietly.

Sandy had heard her. 'You wish I was your mum. I feel honoured.' She paused.

The room felt so silent, so very silent. Two people, from different generations, connecting across the years. To Jodie it felt safe. She felt safe. She felt strangely at home, a kind of calmness that had sort of crept up on her in the last couple of minutes. Sandy was also aware of the silence, and of her wanting to respond to Jodie in ways that were going to help her come to terms with what she was experiencing.

'I'm going to speak to her. I think I want to head off and do it now. It just feels right, that it is something that I need to do.'

Sandy nodded. 'OK, you feel in the right place in your self to say what you want to say, yeah?'

'I do. Yes, I'll head back. Mum will be home now.'

Sandy agreed. What Jodie was experiencing had emerged from their encounter that afternoon. It was very real for her, for them both. She wanted to allow Jodie to hold what she was feeling and to take it with her. But she also wanted to point out that she might want to just take care of herself, going back out into a noisy world. She highlighted this. Jodie listened and agreed to bear this in mind.

Sandy felt comfortable with what Jodie wanted to do. She felt safe. She had no sense of a need to say anything about how safe she felt. And she didn't want to undermine her in any way. She trusted that Jodie's own inner process had brought her through a realisation about change, growing up, the future. No doubt it would still arise, but she wanted to trust that Jodie had developed a resource in herself this session to find a way through it. She hoped that Jodie's mother would listen and respond helpfully. Maybe this will bring them closer together.

Sandy might have been left feeling very anxious still and, had this been the case, she may well have voiced this. But it is not in her experience and it would therefore be inauthentic to introduce something that she thinks Jodie should hear but which isn't being experienced for her as pressing. This kind of situation arises increasingly in a world where healthcare professionals have to constantly (or so it seems) be mindful of risk. Yet it can stifle trust – one of the most valuable therapeutic attitudes that the therapist can hold towards their clients – when it is genuinely present. The person-centred counsellor will seek to be true to their own experiencing.

Points for discussion

- How are you left feeling after the session?
- Should Sandy have voiced concerns for Jodie's safety? If so, why? If not, why not? Link this to person-centred theory.

- How do you think Sandy handled Jodie's comment about wishing Sandy was her mum? How would you have handled this? What other possible responses might she have made?
- Consider and discuss the different kinds of silence that can arise within counselling sessions.
- Evaluate the counsellor's application of a person-centred way of working in this session.
- Write your own notes for the session.

CHAPTER 7

Counselling session 7: Jodie has spoken to her mum, relationship changes

Jodie had arrived early. She had caught an earlier bus. She felt she had so much to talk about, and she sort of hoped that maybe she might get seen sooner, and perhaps have a longer session. It had been a good week; she had had a really good heart-to-heart with her mum who – she had been amazed – had listened and shown so much caring. By the time she had got back from the previous session, her anxieties had returned, and she had seen her mother in the front room with a magazine. She had gone in and said where she had been, and that she wanted to talk about something.

Her mother had looked surprised at first, but had put the magazine down. Jodie then started to tell her about the session and about her fears and somehow everything had sort of come out in a bit of a rush, and she had ended up in tears again. But her mum had been so good. She had listened and, well, in the end Jodie had ended up curled next to her on the sofa. She couldn't remember when she had felt that close.

The next day they went shopping together, with Karen, and somehow things felt so different between them. She felt, well, she wasn't sure what she felt, but it had felt good. And it was something she wanted to make sense of today.

Sandy came out and Jodie went into the counselling room and described what had happened. Sandy was pleased, and so appreciated how wonderful it must have been for Jodie to connect in the way that she had with her mother. After she had spoken about it for a while, Jodie suddenly added, 'You know, none of this could have happened without you. I left here feeling so calm, so ready to speak to Mum. I just knew I had to.'

'I'm really pleased it has worked out, Jodie. Must make you feel, well, I guess I'm not sure how it makes you feel, but it gives me a warm feeling inside.' Sandy was being genuine.

> Sandy has stopped herself from saying that she understands how the client feels. 'I understand' is not a helpful way of conveying understanding, particularly as the truth is that until the client has really conveyed what they are feeling, the counsellor has no idea, and even though they may hear the client's words, it does not mean that the meanings the client ascribes to those words are the same as the counsellor's.

'I feel like, I don't know, it's weird but it's like she's my mum again. That's daft 'cos I know she is, but somehow she just feels like Mum. I can't explain it.'

'Seems like a good explanation to me, but maybe you are unsure about how you are describing what you feel?'

'It's like we've connected and I just kind of feel different.'

'Different?'

'Oh, this will sound silly . . .' She paused. Sandy waited. Jodie continued, 'It's like it's not just that she's my mum again, but I feel kind of like her daughter again? Does that make sense?'

'Yeah, what I am hearing is like your relationship has changed and she is back as a mum to you and you a daughter to her.'

Yes, thought Jodie, yes, that's it. 'Yeah, you've got that right. Yeah . . .' Jodie sat and thought about the way Sandy had worded what she had said. It wasn't quite what she had said, but it really had just made an impact on her.

'That feels good, what you just said. You know, I think I've kind of allowed her to be my mum again.' She paused again.

Sandy was nodding.

'It's me that's changed, isn't it? Mum hasn't changed, but I have. I've let her see parts of me that I kind of kept hidden – hidden, I guess, from everyone. The scariness, I didn't dare show that, not to her, or to my friends. That would be bad for my credibility. But it's me. It's me, isn't it?'

'That scariness is a part of you and you have allowed your mum to see it.'

'I wonder what will happen next?'

Sandy was unsure what Jodie was meaning. 'You've lost me; you wonder what will happen next?'

'With me and Mum. I hope it stays like this.'

'Mhmm, you really want it to stay like it is now between you and Mum?'

'I do. It feels good.'

The thought struck Sandy that in one sense Jodie could be letting go of a need to assert herself and her independence in her relationship with her mother, growing away from the need to be what in the past seemed quite combative and hostile. It could be a sign of maturing. At the same time, it could be a flight back into daughterhood as a way of avoiding facing the future and the reality of growing up. Back to the notion of the development of configurations within Jodie, she thought. It seems like her sense of herself as a daughter has reasserted itself, yet maybe now it has developed within itself, or is developing, fresh attitudes and behaviours to those previously present as part of this configuration.

'Good to feel the way you do now.'

'Yes.' As she said this, though, Jodie was aware that all was not totally well. She did still feel worried about the future, but she felt a little more, no much more, settled in herself about it.

The session continued after a short silence, which had felt quite comfortable to them both. Jodie said that she was really struggling to think about what else to say. She talked about school, and the fact that the summer break was fast disappearing. That she didn't know what she wanted to do when she left, but she guessed she would do her A levels. She realised this wouldn't be easy; she hadn't been the best pupil in the school, other things had been more important, but now it felt different. She was still confused by it all. Sandy had empathised with the presence of this confusion for Jodie.

'I just don't seem to be me, but I am me, but then I'm not. It's like things that were important, I mean, I'm not really thinking of them so much.'

'Some things are losing their importance to you.'

'Not just things. I've seen Em, but not Ally, who's away this week. We went to the cinema, and it was good, I enjoyed it, but I'm different, and I kind of feel good about it at home, but it feels really odd when I'm out.'

'So, the feelings are comfortable at home, yeah?'

'But not when I'm out, well, not when I'm with friends. I feel sort of distant from them. And I don't like that. I feel out of it, somehow, just not where they're at. And I don't know how to get back there, and I kind of want to, and I don't want to, but I think I do really.'

> Sandy had empathised with the comfort at home but not the feeling odd when out. Jodie is quick to repeat that, indicating that it is important to her and she wants Sandy to hear it.

'Sort of think you do, but you're not sure?'

'I mean, we've been such good friends for so long, and I guess I want to still be with them.' Jodie stopped and thought about it. She could see them both in her mind's eye, and as ever they were joking around. She missed that, but she also liked how she was at the moment. She just wasn't clear what to do.

'My sense is that you want to be as you are, and spend time with your mum, and doing your own thing, and you also want to be with Em and Ally as well.' Sandy felt an urge to add, 'And you can do both', but she wanted this to be Jodie's realisation if it was to emerge.

Jodie nodded. She kind of knew she wanted both, and yet that seemed to be quite a challenge. 'I guess there's such a difference, and I'm kind of different, and I need to be in the right place in myself. Sometimes I want to be on my own; sometimes I want to be with them. But I can't really be sure day to day how I'm going to feel.' She was feeling concerned that when she came to it, she might not always want to do what she had planned for a day.

Sandy could hear the dilemma. 'You want to be sure that you can do what you want to do, but that's difficult. You don't know how you'll feel day to day.'

As she heard Sandy speak Jodie also realised that this was perhaps unreasonable, that she might sometimes have to compromise. Though that wasn't something she found easy. She was used to doing what she wanted, or reacting against anyone who tried to stop her. All very intense, she thought to herself. 'I guess I need to learn to compromise a bit, but that isn't me, or it hasn't been me.'

'Hard to compromise, doesn't feel like you.'

'But I'm going to have to, I mean, I'm just gonna become some selfish bitch if I don't give a little, and that's how I was and that didn't get me anywhere. I don't want to go back to that. So maybe I need to meet up more with Em and Ally again, but also make sure I have time with Mum, and Karen as well, and just get used to it.'

'Sounds like a way to resolve it, give a bit of time to everyone, stop becoming a selfish bitch, yeah?'

Sandy provides an empathic summary, but ending on the note of 'selfish bitch' adds a certain sharpness to it. However, the risk is that Jodie might hear it as Sandy telling her that she thinks that she is a selfish bitch, which is not what Sandy is trying to communicate. Of course, it could be that at some level Sandy is thinking this and therefore that is the reason for the word order of her response.

Jodie was aware that she did miss the times she was out with her mates. Didn't sound that good, hearing Sandy say 'selfish bitch'. 'But I can't get too heavily into the dope; I really feel I have to say no. Does my head in although it's been a good experience too. But I haven't touched any now for a while and I feel good. Yeah, I guess I don't really need it, but it's been hard to say no when it's around. Well, I never really tried to say "no" much, just joined in, but that isn't me any more. I've changed, and I guess I don't know how I'll be with Ally and Em now, but I don't want to lose what we have. It's been so good for so long.'

'Yeah, though you have changed, you really appreciate what you have together.'

Jodie nodded. 'I do.' Some of the crazy things they'd done came to mind. Yeah, she thought, I need to get out and about as well. She realised how it felt like part of her wanted one thing and part of her wanted another. She tried to explain this. 'You know, it feels like part of me is pulled one way, and another part of me is pulled another way.'

'Different parts pulling in different directions.'

'And they're part of me, aren't they, I mean, and, well, I guess I have different needs. Yeah, I'll get to spend more time with Ally and Em. Haven't been to the cinema for a while, or just hung around, joking about. I've kind of got a bit serious recently, haven't I?'

'Mhmm. I guess you have.'

'And that's OK, but I don't only want to be serious. That's really important. I kind of feel I could slide into that and, well . . .' She thought for a moment. 'But then I haven't been serious all the time, with Mum, we've had some laughs. But it kind of feels different, different to laughing with Em and Ally. It's weird.' She shook her head, aware of how complicated it could all seem. She wondered how Sandy coped with it all. 'You must get confused all the time with what you do. Why do you do it?'

Sandy experienced what Jodie had said as a direct question demanding an answer, not an exploration of her need to answer the question. Young people were more direct, and she was sensitive to that.

'To make a difference.' Sandy was being totally honest in her response.

Jodie smiled. 'Well you've made a difference with me. I'm not who I was when I came in here that first time.'

'Thanks, and you've made a difference to yourself as well.' As she said it a quote from Carl Rogers was in her head.

'Individuals have within themselves vast resources for self understanding and for altering their self-concepts, basic attitudes, and self directed behaviour; these resources can be tapped if a definable climate of facilitative psychological attitude can be provided.' (Rogers, 1980, p. 115)

'I'm aware that there isn't much of the school holidays left and I'm not sure about being able to still see you when I'm back at school, and I'm also wondering whether I kind of need to. I mean, I feel like I've changed a lot, and it's been really helpful, and I do like coming here now, but it is in the daytime.'

'Is it because of the daytime that you are wondering about stopping, or you feel you've got what you want from counselling?'

Jodie thought about it. 'Well, I guess I kind of feel I've got what I need. I mean, I didn't know what I needed when I first came, I was marched here by my mum, you know. At the time I didn't like it, hated her for it, but she was right. Hard to admit it, but she was.'

'So how many more weeks do you have off school? Also, you need to know I'm away at the beginning of September for a week.'

'Somewhere nice, I hope.'

Sandy smiled. Whenever you mention going away clients seem to want to know where. Self-disclosure. Why do we make such a big thing about it? Some counsellors want to analyse the client's motivation to the point that they may be put off ever asking a question again. What's that about? Counsellor being over-defensive? Her attitude was that direct questions generally deserved direct answers so long as that answer did not end up being the focus in the session. 'Yes, I'm getting away and hoping for some sunshine.'

'Sounds good. Where?'

'Oh, Greece. But that's me; what about you and what you want to do with the sessions we have? We have next week, then I'm away.'

Jodie thought about it and decided that she felt she could stop. She said this and Sandy suggested that maybe Jodie could think about what she wanted from that final session, what she felt would be helpful to her.

> She did not make suggestions herself, like using it to reflect on the counselling and what it had achieved, and what goals Jodie felt she had for herself. That would have been directive and she wanted Jodie to connect with and voice her own needs.

'I guess see what happens this week, and maybe look ahead a little. I expect I'll have seen Ally and Em before then and it would be good to talk about that.' She stopped as she felt a wave of emotion. 'And it'll be hard ending this too. But I can feel that there's a pull again, part of me wanting to move on and another part wanting to stay here where it feels sort of safe. I like it here.'

Sandy was aware of experiencing feeling curious as to what it was she liked about being here, but she knew that while some might say that you voice this because you are experiencing it – what she termed *pseudo-congruence* – this was not the meaning of congruence that she understood to be such a key aspect of person-centred counselling.

> Being congruent does not mean you have to keep saying what you are feeling. It does not give free licence to anything being said because you are experiencing it. This is a fundamental fact. Congruence is an attitude of being, a condition in which the counsellor can actually experience what is present for them, and to be able to appreciate within that experiencing what is present in response to being in relationship with the client, and what is simply their own stuff having little or no relevance to the session.

'Pulled in different directions again. Want to move on, but it feels safe here.'

'But I can't stay here forever. No, let's have a final session next week and then back to school. I guess I could get back in touch if I needed to?'

'Sure, you can self-refer back in. We cannot guarantee how quickly we'll get to see you, but you can refer back if you feel the need to. I guess I have to say though that it would kind of need to be drug-related, given that's our remit.' Oh shit, thought Sandy as she heard herself say this, I hope that doesn't give her a reason to use. No, that's not where Jodie's at.

'You looked lost for a moment.' Jodie had noticed the change in Sandy's expression. She'd looked momentarily horrified.

Sandy knew it was a moment to be transparent. No point in saying anything other than what she experienced. The last thing Jodie needed was to experience her counsellor, who she had learned to trust, suddenly coming across as evasive. 'It was what I said. I guess I suddenly had the thought that you might go and use something to get to be able to come back, and I know that that's silly. I don't believe that's you, but the thought was there. I now feel I want to apologise for having had that thought, but I also need to acknowledge it was there.'

'That's OK. You're right, but I don't think I'd do that. You never know though! No, seriously, the way I feel at the moment, I don't want to start using anything much. Not even sure how I feel about alcohol at the moment either. But, well, we'll see. Thanks for being honest, though. Somehow that means a lot.'

'If I can't be real with you, how can I honestly expect you to be real with me, you know? I know it's a bit of a cliché, "get real", but in a way that is what it's all about. I just prefer to think of it in terms of being authentic, being openly myself.'

Jodie was listening to what Sandy was saying and it was making her think about herself. 'I guess that's what I've been with Mum, isn't it? Been more real, more, what did you say . . . ?'

'Authentic?'

'Yeah, and it does feel good.' Her thoughts went to Em and Ally. 'Now I've got to be authentic with Em and Ally too. And somehow that feels like it'll be more difficult, and I'm really surprised to hear myself say that. I mean, when I came here, the idea of being real with my mum – well, I guess I thought I was being. But I wasn't really. And I thought I was being real with my mates, but now I can see I wasn't, at least, I wasn't being the me that I am now.'

'You weren't being the you that you are now, couldn't be that with them.'

'And I need to be. Yeah, get real. I can see myself carrying that in my head, you know. Probably bore the shit out of everyone saying it, but it feels good, feels where I need to be.'

Sandy had noticed the time, a few more minutes left of the session. She mentioned it.

'Yeah, OK, so, go and get real, that's my mission for the week. But really real, not selfish-bitch real! That just came into my head.' Jodie grinned. So did Sandy. She loved the way young people could just cut through the complexity sometimes and just come up with a few words that seemed to sum so much up.

'Yeah, go for it.'

The session ended with them agreeing the time for the next and final counselling session. Jodie headed off, and Sandy sat down to write her notes and reflect on what she wanted to take to supervision from the last few sessions with Jodie.

Points for discussion

- Evaluate the effectiveness and accuracy of Sandy's empathic responses.
- How appropriate was Sandy's self-disclosure regarding her holiday? What are your boundaries for self-disclosure?
- Reflect on the impact of Sandy's transparency towards the end of the session.
- Define congruence in your own words.
- The sessions are coming to an end. Do you feel that this is timely? What might be the pros and cons of continued counselling at this time?

CHAPTER 8

Supervision 2

'I want to spend a little time on Jodie, but not too long as I have other clients I need to talk about as well.'

'So, do you want to split the time for each client, or just go with the flow?'

'Go with the flow. I haven't a lot to say, really want to check in with her more than anything else, and to talk about how we are working towards an ending to coincide with the end of the school holidays.'

Courtney felt a sense of surprise.

'You look surprised.'

'I'd kind of imagined that the sessions would go on longer, but I don't know why. Just a sense that I had somehow. Oh well, so, working towards an ending. How is that for you?'

'It sort of feels timely, I mean, with the school holidays ending soon. And it feels like she has done a piece of work on herself in a way, making a lot of changes. She's on much better terms with her mother. She suddenly got in touch with fears of growing up, and she really was terrified, and she decided to talk to her mum about it, which I think was really courageous.'

'Did you tell her that?'

Sandy stopped and thought back. 'No, I don't think I did. I really should have done. I mean, I do recognise the risk she took, that her mum might not have listened or dismissed it in some way. You're right. I saw it more in terms of risk than her courage. It would have been a real act of prizing, wouldn't it? And I missed it.'

'Maybe that's something you could say in the final session if you are reviewing things.'

'Yes. You're right. And it isn't that I need to say it; I'm aware now that I want to say it. And maybe I will if it kind of feels right during the session, sort of fits in with what is being said. But I'm intrigued that it didn't happen in the session.'

'Any thoughts?' Courtney trusted Sandy to reflect for herself on her own process on these kinds of occasion.

'I think I was probably so pleased for her, and she wasn't kind of presenting it as a courageous thing to do, that it was never really there to empathise with.'

'Yeah, that happens. We can get so centred in our own feelings for the client and what they have done . . .'

Sandy thought about that comment. Had she been centred in her own feelings? Had she lost connection with Jodie, if only momentarily? What had she said when Jodie had first mentioned it? She thought back. 'I said something about feeling really pleased for her. That was just so weak, wasn't it. "Oh, I'm so pleased for you." Yuck. Where was I? Jodie was talking about how good it had felt. I somehow didn't tune in to her.'

'Mhmm. Couldn't tune in to her feeling good about the change in her relationship with her mother.'

Sandy went quiet. 'Ouch.'

Courtney raised his eyebrows as if to say, 'Yes?'

Sandy sighed. 'My mother. Dammit. You never really get away from your parents, do you? Work through issues, but they're always around somewhere, waiting to catch you out. I never really did get to know my mother much as a child. Never really had the kind of relationship that it seems Jodie is creating.'

Sandy sat for a moment. She heard Courtney's response, 'Never had with your mother what Jodie has with hers.'

Sandy shook her head, aware that her own feelings were surfacing. Shit, she thought, I'm still feeling that loss. She placed her hand across her mouth, supported her elbow and leaned back into the chair with a sigh. 'Part of me still wants that. I thought I'd come to terms with it, and accepted it. But I haven't, have I?'

'That how it feels, you still want what Jodie has?'

Sandy nodded. 'Yes. I don't get on well with my mother, never have really. Always seem to end up arguing about things. She has to have it all her way. I still can never get anything right. She doesn't believe in therapy, and I do still get the odd comment about having a proper job, that she didn't have to have counsellors, just got on with it. More's the pity, I think, maybe she'd have turned out a bloody sight better.' Sandy was aware of the rising energy inside her.

Courtney had noticed it too. 'All fired up, huh? Maybe she'd have turned out a bloody sight better.' He kept with her feelings, and allowed her the space to flow with her experiencing.

Sandy could feel her jaw tighten as she took another deep breath. 'Yeah. Aaagh. Well, I'm glad to be aware of it anyway, and it will help me self-monitor. It's so easy to slide into complacency, to think you've resolved issues. But no, OK, I can appreciate what's happened. I'll be a little more self-aware from now on when Jodie talks of her mother.'

'Mhmm, and a little more congruent?'

'Yeah. I need to be open to my experiencing and to really know what it is and where it is coming from. In this case it wasn't that I was left feeling something that was mine which got in the way, but more I was left not feeling ... No, that's not right, is it? I wasn't feeling. I wasn't feeling a sense of what Jodie would have been feeling, about how good it had been. I have to watch my empathy towards her positive experiences with her mother. Yeah, I have to watch that.'

'Mhmm. So how do you experience being with Jodie now? What's the quality of your empathy like?'

'Well, before our conversation just now, I would have said really good. I have a real sense of her growing, or rather, more growing up I suppose. She's thinking more and in touch with different aspects of herself. She talks of spending more time at home, of being with her mother and feeling less drawn to be with her two mates, Em and Ally. Yet she's also not wanting to really lose the relationship with them either.'

'Yeah, thanks for the summary, and I still wonder what the quality of your empathy is like?'

Courtney has sensed that Sandy is having difficulty connecting with this aspect of her relationship with Jodie, and he feels it is important for her to explore this, to clarify it. If her empathy isn't there, Jodie is not going to experience a crucial aspect of the 'necessary and sufficient conditions', and as Sandy's supervisor he feels, and has, a responsibility to ensure that Jodie receives this.

Sandy nodded. 'You're right. I'm struggling to connect with it. How do I feel being in relationship with Jodie, or Jode as she prefers to be called. Funny that, just saying Jode sort of changes things. Makes her feel more alive somehow. Jode. It feels kind of exciting, yeah, like watching something growing. It's really satisfying being with her. I feel like I am nourishing her, like I'm giving her what she needs to grow? And yet I know that I can't make her grow, just create a climate of relationship which will encourage her to discover more of herself and greater authenticity. Yeah, authenticity, it feels like we are getting progressively more real with each other – except for me not being able to empathise with her about her mother. Damn. She's growing and I might get in the way. And I can't do that. OK, I'll really be aware of myself, but not to the point of not listening. But I have to be focused when she talks about her mother. If I'm still struggling I'll take it to personal therapy, Courtney, and have another go at clearing it, or whatever. I'm aware of the time and I have a couple of new clients I want to talk about as well today. Is that OK?'

Courtney smiled, and Sandy knew why. He wasn't going to tell her, but leave it for her to decide. 'OK, I know, I'm a grown up and can make my own judgements. I feel what I'm suggesting is appropriate. And I'm really glad it came up. It's just so easy for something to get in the way, and it doesn't feel like it at the time, and it may not have had any impact on Jodie, but it might have done. She might have connected more with her own positive feelings, maybe more deeply, who knows, and that may have been therapeutically valuable. But the opportunity was lost.' She shook her head.

'You're shaking your head.'

'Well, it makes me appreciate the importance of this kind of supervision, where I can be given space to explore and where you can respond in the way that you do, holding me in uncomfortable places, or areas of myself I have lost sight of. It's so important when working with people in a therapeutic way and I just wish people appreciated this. I just get pissed off when people say, "Supervision? Don't you know how to do your job?" They just have no idea. Sorry, getting fired up again. I just feel that people do not understand our profession, and maybe that's about us not going out and explaining it, and maybe I have to take responsibility in that too.'

Courtney smiled. 'Yeah, you touch on some important things, Sandy, dear to my own heart as well. And I'd really like to explore this, and I know that that's because it's an area that gets me going too, but you have two new clients . . . ?'

Points for discussion

- Did Sandy raise all the issues from the previous sessions that required supervision?
- What are your views on the role and value of supervision in other professions?
- Names can be so important. Do the names 'Jodie' and 'Jode' conjure up a different sense of the client for you?
- The issue of the counsellor being too centred in their own feelings to sense what the client is experiencing and communicating is important. What areas of feeling might you experience that would block you from hearing and empathising appropriately with a client?
- Evaluate the supervision session in terms of Courtney's responses.

CHAPTER 9

Counselling session 8: saying no to pills and appreciating her mum

Jodie was a few minutes late and apologised as she came into the room. 'Damn bus, just seemed determined to go slow today. And so much traffic. Anyway, I've made it.'

'Yes, sounds a bit stressful.' Sandy wanted to give Jodie an opportunity to talk about this should she wish to.

'Yeah. Anyway. So, I want to tell you about my week. I know it's the last session but something happened that I feel really good about, but also a bit mixed up with as well. I kind of want to make sense of it, you know?'

'OK. Mixed up and wanting to make sense of what happened. Where do you want to start?'

> Very businesslike. Quick, empathic reflection and an offering to the client to choose where to begin.

'Well, after last time, you know, we talked ... well I talked about getting back to seeing Em and Ally more. And, well, I did. We went out a couple of times and then over the weekend, and I kind of had fun, you know, but I also felt sort of different still. I mean, at times I really was me again, you know, messing around and stuff, and just having some fun. But at other times, I just kind of felt myself drifting and feeling like I wanted to head back home.'

'Mhmm.' Sandy didn't get a chance to say anything else; Jodie was continuing.

'And then on Saturday we went to this party, and that was good, we were dancing and stuff and I met this guy and we kind of spent time together and danced and stuff, and that was really good. And, well, Ally had these pills and she wanted me to have one. Said her brother had given them to her, said she and Em had had them the previous Saturday and it had been really good. They'd really given them both a boost and it was great, and they wanted me to have one. And I really didn't want to. I mean, I really knew that I didn't want to. But I didn't know what to do.'

Sandy felt herself make the assumption that it was ecstasy, though she knew it might be something else. Anyway, she wanted to allow Jodie to carry on with her story.

Ecstasy comes in tablet form, various colours, and can leave people feeling they are full of energy, hence it has become known as a 'dance drug'. It can have a mild hallucinogenic effect, giving people the sensation of being 'spaced out', and leaves the user thinking that everyone is their friend. But it can also leave people feeling panicky. As the drug wears off the user can feel really tired but actually find it difficult to sleep. People have died from first use, and it is dangerous when used to keep the user dancing in hot environments, as they can overheat, which can be fatal. There is a distinct possibility of depression and other mental health complications later in life from heavy use. The pills can also be of varying quality and include other substances, enhancing their problematic impact.

'So you were faced with them encouraging you to take a pill, and you really didn't want to.'

Jodie shook her head. 'I just knew I didn't want to. I mean, the party had been good and there wasn't any alcohol around. Mark's parents – it was at his house – had organised soft drinks and food and stuff, and had really made sure no alcohol was there. And I felt OK with that. But I was really surprised with Ally. She kept saying no one would know, that it's not like smoking dope, no one can smell it in the air. In the end I took it, but I didn't have it, just said thanks and headed back on to the dancefloor. I later threw it away. I just didn't want it, didn't need it. I was enjoying myself. But it really left me feeling, shit, just so confused. Kind of stayed with me, you know?'

'Yeah, preyed on your mind.'

'I really felt that somehow Em and Ally were heading in a different direction to me. And you know the thought that struck me later, much later, was that a few weeks ago I probably would have swallowed that pill, whatever it was. I'd have just done it because, well, you do what your mates do. But I'm not there any more. That incident really made me aware of that.'

'You're just not in the same place as Em and Ally, but you would have been a few weeks back.'

Sandy might have also mentioned the fact that Jodie didn't take the pill, but rather she has focused on the sense that Jodie is in a different place and has held her on that contrast. This has enabled Jodie to focus on change in herself. Of course, this could be seen as directive, although Jodie remains free to bring the focus back to the issue around whether or not she would have taken the pill offered to her if she had not had counselling.

Distinguishing whether or not a response has been directive can be subtle. Plus, one has to take into account the counsellor's experience in the moment, which may be that something about the way a client has spoken has communicated where their own emphasis is.

'Coming here has changed me in ways I wasn't expecting. And it's hard to explain why, I mean, you just sit and listen and tell me pretty much what I've told you. But somehow it's made me think, made me question myself. Something else in me has kind of, I don't know, sort of grown somehow. It's weird, but it's happened and I'm sure that if I hadn't come to counselling I'd have swallowed that pill on Saturday. And I just don't want to go there.'

'Mhmm. It's a place that you just don't want to go to, but a few weeks back you probably would have done.'

Jodie nodded. 'And that's scary. I mean, you know, that's scary. I'm not wanting to get into that, into Es, you know. I mean, I know there's all kinds of things said about them, and some say it's OK and others that they're dangerous, and I just get confused by it all. But what I do know is that I feel good these days and I really don't need it. I really don't need it.'

'That sounds clear, feeling good and you don't need it.'

'But I'm really concerned for Em and Ally. I mean, they don't seem to care. It's still all a big laugh for them, but it isn't for me, not any more, not that stuff. I mean, what's her brother going to give her next, you know? I spoke to Ally on the phone on Sunday. She wasn't feeling too good. I said that I was really concerned, that I hadn't taken it, and didn't want to and really felt she needed to think about what she was doing. She told me not to make a fuss, that she was OK, she was going to do what she wanted to do and that if I didn't like it I could fuck off.' As she spoke, Jodie could feel herself becoming more and more emotional. Tears had welled up in her eyes. 'I really care about her, Sandy, I mean, I love her to bits, she's been part of my life for so long, but I think I'm losing her, or that's the risk. I don't want to go where she's going. And I don't know about Em. I haven't spoken to her. I kind of feel Ally will drag her into it.' Jodie paused. 'I don't want to go there, I really don't.'

'Really concerned about Ally and Em, what they are doing, where it will lead, and feeling that you don't want to go there.'

Sandy is seeking to show or check out her empathic understanding. She is not saying a lot, but keeping her responses focused, and it is allowing or enabling Jodie to explore her own thoughts and feelings and to connect more deeply with what is present for her.

As Jodie listened to Sandy the tears finally welled up over her eyelids. She felt suddenly so sad, and so alone. Her best friends, both starting to dabble around with other drugs. She knew that she didn't want to go down that path. But she also knew that she didn't want to lose her friends. She felt awful, unable to know what to do for the best.

'And it makes me worry about going back to school, I mean, it's all going to be different. I'll probably be on my own, and I really don't know quite what I'm going to do. It'll feel tough, I know it will. And I can't really talk to mum about this, I mean, if I mention drugs to her she'll go crazy, start phoning up their parents and stuff, and I don't want that. It'll be awful. But I kind of feel I need to talk to someone about it, you know?'

Sandy was wondering about whether she could juggle her own availability to carry on seeing Jodie, if only to offer her something while she acclimatises to being back at school. She thought about the school counsellor, if there was one. She wanted to explore options, particularly if this was to be the last session.

Sandy is realistically concerned and is hearing Jodie express her need to have someone to talk to. She therefore introduces her concern and makes an offer to extend the counselling. It is therefore introduced in response to the presence of the core conditions: her concern and caring for Jodie, her empathic understanding of Jodie's expressed need, and her congruent experience of feeling an urge to offer her more that is emerging from their therapeutic contact.

'I'm kind of wondering about revisiting what you might get by way of further support through all of this. I mean, I know we decided last week to end, and that's fine, but I wonder whether you can come here after school?'

'Yeah, I could, but not in school uniform, you know? I mean, I'd have to go home and change and come back. Couldn't get here before five o'clock and even that might be difficult sometimes.'

Sandy could offer that, she could reorganise her timing, but it would have to be on a different day. She explained this and they spent some time discussing whether there might be a possibility for one day during the week. It turned out that Thursday was the most likely day. Sandy also mentioned the school counsellor as another option, but Jodie didn't want to do that. 'Everyone knows. You have to leave lessons and stuff. No, I'd rather carry on coming here. Just to get me through going back to school, anyway. Can you do that?'

They agreed that they would set up a couple more appointments on Thursdays at 5.00pm, or as soon as Jodie could get there, after Sandy was back from her break. Sandy realised she felt more at ease. And Jodie was really happy. Somehow, going back to school didn't seem so difficult.

There was still quite a bit of the session left and Sandy asked Jodie how she wanted to use the time.

'I guess I want to ask some questions about different things. I mean, well, I suppose I'd like some information, you know, on Es and stuff. I'd like to take something for Em and Ally as well. I just feel that if something happened, well, that I hadn't at least tried to help them understand.'

'OK, we have some leaflets geared up for young people, and I can give you some copies before you go.' Sandy paused, and then returned to the tone of what Jodie had been saying. 'You really care about them, don't you?'

Sandy has managed, very effectively, to acknowledge the need for information and offered a practical response to that, but has sought to not let it interrupt the therapeutic flow, bringing the focus back on to Jodie's concerns for Em and Ally.

'I do. I mean, I know things are a bit difficult between us at the moment, but, well, we've been through a lot together, you know, and that means something. They're kind of like sisters to me. But I also realise that maybe I've spent so much time with them I haven't made other friends. Maybe I have to think about that as well. Ally really was nasty on the phone when she told me to "fuck off", and I really don't know why she was like that. Feels like she's changed somehow. Or am I just seeing her differently? I don't know. But I don't want to lose their friendship; they've been really important to me.'

Sandy nodded and acknowledged how important they had been, aware that Jodie had been talking in the past tense and making a point of empathising with that.

'I think Mum will be pleased that we are having a few more sessions. She seemed a little hesitant when I told her we were planning to end today. She asked about phoning on my behalf, but I had said no. At the time, I really did feel OK about it, but after last weekend, well, I'm glad we can have a few more. I don't think I want lots, but just in case things are difficult. I really appreciate it, you know?'

'Yeah, things changed with the incident at the weekend and it's good we have been able to work something out. We'll see how things are next time and take it from there, yes?'

Jodie nodded. 'That feels good.'

'Mhmm. Good feeling.'

'Sort of reassuring. Like, I'm not really on my own. In fact, with things different at home and with you, I feel like I have a lot of support. It's so good to feel listened to and taken seriously. That's something so new for me, but it feels so good. I wish ...' Jodie didn't finish the sentence. What she wanted to say sounded daft.

'You wish.'

'I was going to say, wish I'd had this earlier. But then, I don't think I'd have got as much out of it.'

'Mhmm, it feels like it would have been good, but you're unsure as well.'

'I keep trying to think about what exactly has happened. I mean, yes, you've listened and we've talked about stuff, but, I mean, OK, I have been upset at times, but, well, I guess saying about my fears of growing up, that was really important, and that somehow led me to talk to Mum, and things really accelerated then. But I'd been spending time on my own and thinking about things. And it is still all very scary, you know. But somehow I don't feel so alone with it.'

'Not so alone?' Sandy wanted to just encourage Jodie to expand on this but to do this in such a way that she felt she had been heard.

'Yeah, it's like I haven't got to bottle it up any more? I was, but hadn't really thought I was. But now I can talk to Mum, and to you. And it helps with how it is with Mum now, and that makes it easier to think of ending here sometime. It's like I still have someone.' She was nodding her head.

'It's important, isn't it, to have someone to feel you can turn to.' Sandy was sensing the importance of this. It really was crucial. Without someone to talk to, Jodie could be less resilient to all kinds of temptations, particularly the drugs. But she had a more secure sense of family now. Sandy was also aware of a creeping wonder about her father, who Jodie never talked about. But she respected this. No doubt she had her reasons. Perhaps he didn't figure in her life much. Maybe Karen had a closer relationship with him. Sandy realised she was drifting into her own speculation and brought herself back to Jodie in the present.

'Yeah, and it does make such a difference at home. It's less tense, I feel more relaxed. It just feels different. We do stuff together. It's become really, really important to me.' As she spoke Jodie could feel the tears welling up in her eyes. Sandy had noticed this too.

'Yeah, it really touches you deeply, Jode.'

Responding to body language can be extremely powerful. The tears in Jodie's eyes have communicated to Sandy how strong her feelings were. They don't convey exactly what the feeling is, but that feelings and emotions are strongly present. Sandy therefore communicates empathic appreciation of this by not referring to a particular feeling or emotion, but simply acknowledges that Jodie has been deeply touched.

Jodie nodded and sniffed, took out a tissue and blew her nose. She took another and dabbed at her eyes. But the tears started to flow. 'I'd be lost without her. I never realised how she could be. Or maybe I'd forgotten. I don't know. But we've sort of become friends. She cares.'

Sandy was listening but she also suddenly remembered that earlier session when Jodie had said something about how she, Sandy, seemed to care, and how she had responded. Yes, even then, feeling cared for and cared about was so important. Then she didn't feel her mother cared. She no doubt did, but Jodie wasn't experiencing it. Now that had all changed. She knew her mother cared, and she felt so much better for it.

'Feeling that care, it's just so important to you.'

Jodie could see her mother's expression when she had told her about how scared she was of the future. She didn't think she would ever forget it. Her mum had had tears in her eyes, and had just reached out to her and held her. It was something that hadn't happened for a while, and she realised how much she had missed it. Sitting there that afternoon, next to her on the settee, it was like ... it was like she had come home. She had become her mother's daughter again, and it had felt good. She could stop trying to be the little miss adult, stropping around the house, always wanting her own way, never wanting to listen to anyone else. She shuddered when she thought of how she had been.

The session continued with a further exploration of Jodie's feelings towards her mother and a reflection on some of her memories, both happy and uncomfortable. Yet she rarely mentioned her father, it was always Mum. She maintained her empathic sensitivity towards what Jodie was telling her.

As the session drew to a close, Jodie suddenly said, 'I don't say much about Dad, of course, but he never really has had much time for me. Always more interested in Karen.' Sandy was immediately struck by the words that Jodie was using.

'More interested?'

'Well, he always seems to spend more time with her, always has right from early on. I don't know why. We've never really got on. He's always busy, working long hours, then he's out at weekends playing golf and, well, he really doesn't seem to spend that much time at home at all. I think in a way my being closer to Mum has been really good for her. I don't think she's really happy. I know I wouldn't be, but that's how they are. They live almost independent lives. I wonder sometimes what keeps them together. It's not that they row or anything. Well, they have disagreements, but nothing more than that. They're just so different.'

Sandy empathised with what Jodie had said, which allowed her to say a little more.

'I suppose I don't really respect him much. He doesn't seem to do much around the house, Mum always has to really nag at him to do anything, and even then, it never gets done. Seems to live in his own world half the time, just doing what he wants. I think Mum's fed up with it but she's never said anything to me. The occasional eyes to the ceiling, or a comment along the lines of 'Well, that's your dad', usually followed by a sigh. He does spend time with Karen, but even that seems to have tailed off. I don't know, I can't really make him out. At times it almost seems like he's not interested in having a family. And then, at other times, he can be there for us, taking us out and stuff. But I'd never really describe him as being *fun*. I don't know.'

'You kind of sound confused by how he is, and it seems your mother is kind of putting up with him?'

Quite a short empathic response, which is responding as much perhaps to *how* Jodie is speaking as it is to *what* she is saying. The comment about her mother putting up with him is not empathic; there is no definite indication from what Jodie has said that that is what her mother is feeling. Maybe this is coming from some other experience of Sandy's: in the past, another client, a friend, who knows? But she is oblivious to it as being something not appearing to be present in Jodies frame of reference.

'Something like that. It's kind of sad, but it's how it is. We all have to make the best of it. But he never really shows much affection. I miss that. I see other dads, and, well, it does make me sad sometimes.' Jodie went quiet and Sandy noticed the atmosphere became more concentrated in the room, often a sure sign of emotions coming to the surface.

'Leaves you with a lot of uncomfortable feelings and emotions, huh?'

Jodie nodded, tears had formed in her eyes and she sniffed. 'I wish he'd be more part of things.' She started to cry but soon began to dry her eyes. 'I guess he is how he is, but it isn't easy for Mum, or for me, and I guess Karen as well.'

'Doesn't make it any easier saying that though.'

Jodie shook her head.

The session was drawing to a close. Jodie had noticed the time a few minutes before. 'Well, I guess it's time to go. I wish he would get close like Mum has. Maybe I'll try to do something about it, or talk to Mum, or something. I don't know what, but you've made me more aware of how uncomfortable it is, and I want to do something about it.'

'It sounds really important to you.' Sandy was experiencing a real sense not so much of desperation, but of that kind of resigned sadness coupled with a sense of hope that maybe it could be better, if only ... but without a sense of what might cause things to change.

'Yeah. Anyway, time to go. I don't want to miss my bus.' Jodie looked at the clock and got up. 'Have a great holiday and see you in two weeks, yeah?'

'Thanks, Jode. Yes. See you then. And good luck with going back to school and, oh, nearly forgot, let's get the leaflets on your way out.'

Sandy stopped by the store cupboard and took three copies of a range of leaflets and gave them to Jodie.

Points for discussion

- When Jodie mentioned being offered ecstasy, what was your reaction? Would you have responded differently?
- What about the brother who is 'supplying'? Would you breach confidentiality on that and, if so, how would you justify it? Imagine it was disclosed in different counselling settings. How might this influence a decision?
- Was Sandy sufficiently empathic throughout the session?
- If Jodie had been, say, five years older, would you as a counsellor have interacted differently with her, and if so, why and how?
- Young people and difficulties with 'best friends' are common. How did Sandy enable Jodie to own what she needed to do?
- While Sandy has been aware that there has been little or no focus on Jodie's father, she has not introduced it. How do you feel about him? Could your feelings affect your ability to accurately empathise with Jodie, or could you stray into sympathy?
- Write notes for this session.

CHAPTER 10

Counselling session 9: back to school, seeking out new friends

'I really have found it difficult.' Jodie sat, looking rather depressed by it all. It was
an expression Sandy hadn't seen on her face for a while. Reminded her of those
early sessions with Jodie slumped in the chair staring ahead of her.
'Mhmm. Difficult.' Sandy kept with the focus Jodie had taken.

Sandy might have said something along the lines of 'More difficult than you
expected', but that would have directed her away from the experience of 'difficulty' and into her expectations, also taking her away from an opportunity
to be with her experiencing in the here and now. The person-centred counsellor tries to be a companion at the client's side, not looking ahead or looking back, but at what the client tells them they are experiencing.

'It just feels all wrong. I'm sort of spending more time with other people. I know
Em and Ally are around but we just don't seem to be in the same space any
more.' She went quiet.
'Yeah, different space but it feels all wrong.'
Jodie sighed. 'I don't know. I guess I miss them, and yet I also know that I don't as
well. But I do really.' She looked up at Sandy. 'It's horrible. I want to say "fuck
off" to both of them, but I don't feel that way, not really, not deep down. I want
to be mates with them again, but I don't want to kind of get into where they're
at any more.'
'Mhmm. Deep down you really want to be with them, but not be with what they're
getting into.' Sandy really felt for Jodie, sitting there looking so miserable.
What was it Courtney had asked her that last supervision session, about the
quality of her empathy? Quick reality check. What was she feeling? Compassion. That was the word. She felt she wanted to reach out from the heart and
share with her in her difficult emotions.

'I know I can't get into that. And I am making some new friends, which is good, and doing different things. Joined in a few activities at lunch-times. There's a theatrical group in the school and I've joined that. They meet up one lunch-time – Mondays. I just know I need to get into different things, and not just hang out in the way Em and Ally do. They don't really say much to me. It's changed so quickly. I just feel a big part of me is missing.'

'And it's a big part that's missing.'

Jodie nodded. 'I just feel lost. I really am surprised. I don't understand how it could all change so quickly. I just don't understand.'

'No, just so hard to understand. Good friends a few weeks back, and now ...'

'Nothing, well, no, not nothing, just feeling,' Jodie sighed and breathed out heavily, 'just feeling lost without them.'

Sandy nodded. 'Yeah, lost without them.'

That was how Jodie felt. Lost. Lost in herself. She'd made the effort to get involved in things at school, and she'd been able to focus in most of the lessons – Em and Ally weren't in all of her classes – but break-times were difficult. She sat thinking about this and just feeling that horrible churning emptiness inside her. She took a deep breath. 'But I can't ...' She stopped. She hadn't really thought through what she was going to say; the words came out but she didn't know what to say next.

'I can't ...?' Sandy sought to empathise and help her to perhaps say what something had stopped her from saying. She used the first person; this could sometimes have a more powerful effect, particularly in this kind of situation.

'I can't imagine how it's going to be. I mean, I can't stay like this, feeling the way I do. I love them to bits, Sandy, but they're making me so miserable.'

'You love them to bits but they make you miserable, and you can't stay feeling like you do but can't imagine the future.'

Jodie shook her head. Can't imagine the future. Can't imagine life without those two by her side. She could feel the water building up inside her eyes, and her throat was suddenly dry and felt like it had a lump in it. She swallowed. 'We've had so many good times together and I guess I just assumed it would carry on. I can't believe that it won't.'

'Mhmm, that it won't carry on.'

Jodie heard Sandy respond. It felt so good to feel she was there, listening, hearing what she was saying. She knew she needed someone to help her through this. She was also talking to her mum about it, and that was good; she'd suggest things they could do together. But somehow it was different here, with Sandy. She sort of listened differently, but she couldn't really describe the difference.

'But I have to get used to it, and maybe things'll change again. Maybe I'm being negative. Maybe it'll blow over. I hope it will. I really hope it will. But I guess until then I have to get on and do different things, and, well, I've got some stuff coming up. Got to do some work experience placements, and I'm thinking about that at the moment. Sometimes that feels really exciting, and at other times it just feels, "What's the point?" Fuck it!' The words came out forcefully, and took Sandy by surprise.

'Fuck it?'

'Well, yeah, I mean I should be excited by it, and I guess I'm feeling a little pissed off that the stuff with Em and Ally is getting in the way of that. Mum's been telling me to live my own life, make the most of the opportunities, and somewhere inside me I know she's right, but then the hurt just hits me again. But I have got to get on, move on, do what I want to do, and then maybe things will change. I can only hope. But it does piss me off as well.'

'Pisses you off that you are hurting when you should be excited? Am I hearing that right?' Sandy wanted to ensure that she was understanding what Jodie was saying.

Communicating empathic understanding is not a matter of being a technique of reflection, although the person-centred counsellor will also reflect as part of the therapeutic dialogue. There is a difference. Communicating empathic understanding is an attempt to clarify that what the counsellor has heard is what the client was seeking to communicate. It's like saying, 'Do I understand you here?' And it is rooted in a genuine desire to want to understand. If that desire is lacking in a person-centred counsellor, then they probably should seek alternative employment.

   Wilkins (2003) addresses this, indicating that Rogers expressed a certain 'dissatisfaction with the notion of "reflected feelings"' (p. 109), and goes on to highlight the following passage by Rogers: 'I am *not* trying to "reflect feelings". I am trying to determine whether my understanding of the client's world is correct – whether I am seeing it as he or she is experiencing it at this moment. Each response of mine contains the unspoken question "is this the way it is in you? Am I catching just the colour and texture and flavour of the personal meaning you are experiencing right now? If not, I wish to bring my perception in line with yours"' (Kirschenbaum and Henderson, 1990, pp. 127–8).

'Yeah, it's like they're kind of messing things up for me, you know. Like, they ... But it isn't just them, is it? It's me, too.'

'They're kind of messing you up, but it isn't just them, yeah, it's you too?'

Jodie nodded. 'I mean, they don't say much to me, they go off and do their own thing these days. But I kind of, well, I mean, oh shit this is hard.'

'Really hard to put what you feel into words.'

'Yeah, I mean, I want to blame them, and I do. I mean, why do they have to start messing around with drugs? I don't want to go there. I really don't. If they weren't doing that, it would be OK. I know it would.'

'Sounds like you are really blaming them, for getting into drugs more than you. And if it wasn't for the drugs everything would be as it was.'

Yeah, thought Jodie, yeah. That's how it is. 'And I've heard they're messing around with smack now as well. Kind of a rumour among some of the kids that they're smoking it. Probably Ally's fucking brother again. Bastard. I'd like to kick the fucking shit out of him. He's the one that's fucked it all up. I fucking hate him.' Jodie was spitting the words out and looking very tense and angry.

'Makes you fucking angry, you really blame him for it, want to kick the shit out of him.'

A response to be voiced with attitude, reflecting the tone of Jodie, and perhaps enabling her to own even more the depth of her anger.

'Fucking well do. He's ruined our relationship. Shit, I hope he doesn't mess them up. But I don't know what to do. If the school found out they'd be excluded. I don't want that to happen.' Jodie could feel the anger inside her as she spoke.

'Yeah, you really don't want Em and Ally messed up with drugs . . .'

'No, I don't, I still care about them.' She paused. 'Bastard.'

'Yeah, bastard.'

'Fucking bastard.'

Jodie sat in silence for a while. She had been taken aback by the strength of her feelings. She was angry. She'd tried talking to them both at the start of the term, the first day, but they weren't going to listen. Told her she was boring. She hated that. She didn't want to be boring. She had heard them say it at times as well when she'd walked past. She'd ignored them, but it had hurt. She hadn't mentioned this to Sandy. She wasn't sure why. Maybe it just hurt too much.

'Sandy, I want to keep coming here, I mean, you know, make it longer term. It's horrible talking about all this, but it does help. I mean, I don't mean I suddenly feel different, but just being able to talk it through, to be taken seriously. I haven't got friends now that I feel I can talk to like this. Maybe I will in the future, but not at the moment. And Mum, well, she means well, she always tries to make it better. And that's OK. That's good too. But I need somewhere to come and just talk. Can you do that? Can I keep coming?'

'Yes, no problem. It's clearly important to you, Jode, and I'm happy to listen and try and understand what you are saying and going through. It helps the way I listen?'

Sandy realised this was her question, but it felt that maybe this was a moment to reflect on what was happening between them, as Jodie had introduced her wanting to carry on.

Jodie nodded. 'I kind of feel you're honest with me, sort of someone I can rely on. You're kind of reliable, you know, you're there. Oh this must sound like a muddle.'

'How I'm hearing you, Jode, is that you appreciate my being honest with you and being here in a kind of reliable way.'

'It's like, I can talk to you about anything. In fact, I can just talk. I can say what I want. You don't mind what I say or how I say it. And I can just be as well. I don't know, it just feels kind of safe here. It feels good and it is having an effect on me. I know it is. I've changed so much. And it feels good even though it's really difficult. I mean, being here's not difficult but what I feel is difficult. But I really do want to get on. It's a big year this, exams and stuff. I didn't really care much in the past, but now I want to take it all more seriously, I want to get some qualifications. I can see the point to that now. Before, well, didn't give it any thought. Get married, have babies. But I want more than that.'

'That's a lot you've said, you feel safe here, can say what you want. You didn't say this, but it felt to me like you feel accepted for who you are? And you kind of see the future different, wanting more than babies and marriage, yeah?'

As Jodie listened to Sandy she really felt a wave of warmth inside herself. She couldn't really describe it or explain it, but it was sort of reassuring. So often her thoughts could seem muddled in her own head, but when she heard Sandy kind of give them back to her, they always seemed to sound right. She decided to mention this. 'It's weird, but when I think things I can feel really muddled, and I'm not always sure that I'm saying things clearly, but you kind of give it back to me, and it sounds right and good. And it's like, "yeah, that's me", and that's a good feeling.'

'Mhmm, good to feel that "yeah, that's me".' She smiled.

Jodie smiled back. 'That's it, you're doing it again. It's a real skill. I wish I could do that.' Her thoughts left the room for the moment; she could see Em and Ally. 'I wish I could do that for Em and Ally.'

'You'd really like to unmuddle their thinking, yeah?'

Jodie nodded. 'But I can't. I'm learning to accept that, I guess, Or at least, I'm learning that maybe I have to accept it. But I'm not going to give up hope. I'm not going to let a few bad weeks wipe out years of good times. I just have to get free of this horrible, churning emptiness when I think of them, of how it was, of how I thought it would be, and how it actually is.'

Jodie is moving between what she wants for herself and what she wants for others, between feeling good about the counselling sessions, but feeling bad about how it is with Em and Ally. She's really being pulled in different directions in herself, and yet the powerful, warm feeling that she experienced earlier may indicate that she is developing a stronger core to herself, in a sense her own person freed from the 'conditions of worth' that can be such a huge feature in teenage years. Can she become a young person who can accept her needs and not feel driven to conform to social expectation, or the expectations of friends or, tragically in Western society, the advertising media that conditions and exploits young people?

The session continued with Jodie continuing to explore her feelings towards her two friends, and her new-found motivation to get on with school work and to give herself a better chance of more choices for the future. Sandy was aware of feeling increasingly empowered herself as she heard Jodie talk about her hopes and fears, and her determination in spite of her feelings.

The session ended with an agreement to continue the counselling for at least six more sessions, and then review and see what Jodie then felt she needed. She would carry on coming weekly.

Points for discussion

- Jodie has experienced a range of feelings in the session. What enabled her to uncover her anger?
- Assess Sandy's application of the person-centred approach in her counselling both within this session and generally across all the sessions.
- How do you feel about Ally's brother? If a client disclosed to you he was supplying young people with drugs, how would you react? What would you need in order to be able to work with him if he was your client?
- Write notes for this session.
- Based on your experience of the counselling process, write a dialogue for the next session between Jodie and Sandy.

CHAPTER 11

Jodie reflects on her counselling experience

Jodie left the session feeling somehow more whole, more herself, though she couldn't really explain why. Just felt that she could be more of herself with Sandy than with anyone else, and that just felt good. She wished she had a better grasp of language; she kind of sensed that it was more than just good, but it was hard to really put it into words. But she felt lighter in herself as she headed off for the bus. She did feel sorry about Em and Ally, and she was determined to talk to them again if an opportunity arose, and it felt right. She'd noticed that Em had pocketed the leaflet she'd given her while Ally had thrown hers away. So maybe at least Em wasn't so sure about what she was doing. That's a point, she thought, maybe she should try and catch Em on her own some time? Yeah, that felt good, she'd look out for an opportunity. She got on her bus.

As she sat looking out of the window she thought about how she had come a long way in, what, a couple of months. What a summer. She remembered back to that first session, sitting there, her mum waiting outside. It had felt like a sentence, a kind of punishment, banged up with the counsellor for an hour. And yet that had all changed, she had changed, but she still couldn't quite grasp why, other than she felt heard, felt able to be herself, felt accepted for who she was. It felt good. She felt better for it.

The thought ran through her head: maybe it should be compulsory! But she dismissed it. But she wouldn't put counselling down. It had helped her and she was sure it could help a lot of people, particularly the way she had experienced it. Sitting in a room with a stranger, but not a stranger any more. Sitting there talking and being listened to. How could something that simple have such an effect? She knew that she was a little in awe of it. Left her shaking her head.

Shit, she suddenly realised the bus was at her stop. She hurried out of her seat and got off just in time; the conductor was just ringing the bell for the driver to move on. She stood on the pavement, slightly breathless, her heart pounding. So that's what counselling does for you. Makes you nearly miss your bus stop. She was aware she was smiling. No. Not that, not really, but it can help you to catch a different bus, or get off the one you are on that's taking you nowhere. She started to walk home. There were tears in her eyes. It wasn't sadness. She was happy. She was looking forward to listening to the CD she'd bought at the weekend.

Sandy reflects on the therapeutic journey with Jodie

Meanwhile, Sandy was sitting back in the counselling room and was also reflecting on the journey that she and Jodie had taken, and were continuing with. So much change. Not that she had set out to make her change in some particular way, that was anathema to person-centred working. She simply had sought to form a relationship with her, offer her those core conditions, communicate empathic understanding, positive regard and seek to hold a congruent state within herself. She knew she made mistakes. She wasn't the perfect counsellor; who was? And what would that mean anyway? Stupid notion. As far as she was concerned she tried to be herself and to keep with her client. She was in that room, OK, as a counsellor, but primarily as a human being, a person, seeking to relate in a wholesome and healthy way with another person, and often a person in some form of distress.

Jodie had changed through that process. Her relationship with her mother, her relationship with Em and Ally, her relationship with drugs, her relationship with . . . Sandy was suddenly struck by the theme, and it hadn't really forcibly impressed itself on her before now. Relationship change, in so many areas of her life, and with school as well. Even with me, Sandy thought to herself. She pondered on it, and felt herself smiling. Well, yeah, had to really, didn't it, she thought. And then there's the one relationship I haven't mentioned which is, of course, the one that really matters and on which everything else kind of rests: the relationship she has with herself.

Yes, Sandy thought, and she's discovering more of herself. A new determination, a fresh outlook towards school and her future. Of course she's sad about how it is with Em and Ally, but maybe that will change. She seems intent on trying to get back with them somehow, sometime, but it also seems that part of her wants to move on. Parts. That's us as human beings. Made up of parts. Mearns' configurations within the self. Just makes so much sense. And we live through them, and some die away, others develop and grow. No doubt Jodie's current network of configurations will change and in, what, 10, 20, 30 years' time, will probably look very different. But hopefully she will have more self-understanding and will be able to move more freely around within herself, and not get stuck to the point of obsession in one part of herself. If successful therapy is anything, it is surely a means towards greater self-awareness, greater wholeness.

Time to go home. She locked her notes away and headed out. The traffic was building up and she was going to have to queue in a couple of places. Never mind, time for myself, time to relax with that new CD she'd bought earlier in the day, which she had in her bag.

PART 2

Counselling a young person in a school setting

Setting the scene

Simon has been a school counsellor for seven years. Before that he was a youth worker and so has many years of experience of working with young people. He has two afternoon sessions a week in the school, and he has worked there for about 18 months. At first it was difficult; they had not had a counsellor before and there wasn't much appreciation of the importance and nature of counselling confidentiality. They had also had to establish protocols for the kind of issues he would work with, when to consider referring on, ensuring that parents were aware of the counselling service and asking for them to let the school know if they wished to be informed if their child was referred for counselling.

The school has a pastoral care manager and a teacher with the role of child protection officer. Simon had had to refer young people on to her; he wasn't surprised at the number of incidents of sexual abuse, but he knew he had an important professional role in ensuring that the client's need for therapeutic input was preserved, balanced with the need to protect them, or others, from further harm.

He had worked with young people with a range of issues over the years: problems at home, problems with best friends, bullying, stress from school exams, bereavements, substance use and misuse, and the often overlooked but incredibly significant factor of simply growing up and beginning to face the reality of life. Everyone reacted differently and he was often deeply moved by the honest way his clients faced up to and struggled through often incredibly difficult situations.

Clients could self-refer or be referred by a teacher. Nick, the client he was expecting next day, had referred himself. He did not know the background. He had come to him a couple of weeks before asking if he could come and have a chat. He had seemed very subdued but didn't want to say much more. It had come about after Simon had given a talk at a school assembly on the counselling service, what he offered and how anyone could refer themselves.

Simon is married and has two children himself: his son is 19 and at university, his daughter is 15.

CHAPTER 12

Counselling session 1: the client does not attend

The lesson was coming to an end and Nick was watching the clock. The teacher, Mrs Barton, was giving them their homework. He was sort of listening, but his mind was on other things. He had been finding it more and more difficult concentrating. Now he had something else to occupy his thoughts. He had referred himself to the school counsellor and his appointment was now less than ten minutes away.

He had heard the counsellor, Simon was his name, talk about what he did at assembly a few weeks back. He hadn't been completely sure that he wanted to get in touch with him, but, well, things had got worse and he did feel desperate. He wasn't sure what he was going to say. In truth, he wasn't really sure about anything.

The lesson ended. He put his books away and left the classroom, making his way to where he knew the counsellor had his room. Part of him wanted to hurry there, but another part wanted him to slow down. In fact, the latter part didn't really want him to go at all. He just wasn't sure.

The guy had seemed OK, seemed to be someone he felt he could kind of relate to. Very different from his dad, though. Nick felt strangely sad about this. He liked his dad but they didn't have much in common. Life was generally shit at home. He wasn't looking where he was going and nearly bumped into one of the teachers, muttered that he was sorry and continued walking. He sighed.

He felt anxious. What would he talk about? How would he feel? He knew that everyone would know he was going to the counsellor, everyone in the next lesson anyway. They'd want to know why he wasn't there. He wasn't sure how they were going to react. No, he knew how they would react. Probably just make it worse for him. He felt miserable, uncertain. He was walking more slowly now. It was raining outside, grey and cold. But he wasn't noticing. He passed the door where his next lesson would have been and he found himself going back through the door. It was as though his legs had a mind of their own. No, he couldn't see himself sitting there with the counsellor and talking. He didn't like talking anyway, often felt nervous and unsure of himself.

He sat himself down at a desk and waited for the lesson to start.

In the counselling room Simon sat and waited for Nick to arrive. He had referred himself a couple of weeks back, and Simon was expecting him any moment. He enjoyed his work at the school. Sometimes it gave him energy and hope, when he saw the enthusiasm for life displayed by some of the young people he saw, but more often it was difficult. So many problems. So many pressures. He was so grateful not to be a young person in some ways.

Nick was five minutes late and Simon was beginning to wonder if he was going to make it. It was not unusual for his young clients to not always attend. He realised how difficult it could be. Usually if they were going to make it they were pretty good at arriving on time, especially as in this case the counselling session coincided with the start of the next lesson. He glanced at the clock again. He could hear the rain against the window. What a day, he thought, turning his gaze to where the sound was. It was pelting down. The playing fields had standing water on them. His mind drifted back to his own school days, and of having to play football sometimes in the mud. No one was out there now, though.

He brought his thoughts back to the present. Well, it looks like Nick may not be making it. He always sent a note back to the young person to let them know that they could still come another time. He would offer him a time next week. He knew there could be so many reasons. Perhaps he wasn't in school today for some reason? Maybe he had had second thoughts? He knew how difficult some of his clients found it to come along. So many fantasies about what counselling would be like. He had tried to lay some of these to rest in that assembly he had taken a few weeks back, and he hoped his leaflet presented counselling in a fairly relaxed and informal way. But what he couldn't easily get around was that he was an adult, and children so easily learned attitudes towards adults that would make it harder for them to come along and talk openly about their problems.

He sat for a while longer before deciding that he would take out a journal that had arrived that morning. He'd make himself a coffee if Nick hadn't arrived in a few more minutes, and then write out a note to him, saying he was sorry that he hadn't made it but that he would be happy to see him next week. And he wanted to say as well that he appreciated how difficult it could be to come to counselling and that he was there for whenever Nick felt ready to come along.

Counselling session 2: working with silence and the struggle to speak

Nick had received the note from the counsellor the following day. What struck him immediately was that it didn't sound like he was being told off for not attending. Like it seemed OK. That wasn't what usually happened. Late for a lesson, or not turn up, and you were in trouble. But that wasn't what he experienced reading Simon's note.

It had left him thinking and feeling that, well, maybe he would give it a go. It had been a bad week as well and now it was coming up to that time again and he felt this week that he really had to attend. He still felt very anxious about it, and unsure what he was going to say, or anything really. But he felt he couldn't go on the way things were.

> Simon has managed to convey acceptance of Nick's decision not to attend, which has had the effect of challenging Nick's expectations. He is curious, not sure what to make of it. It has contributed to encouraging him to attend next time.

The sunshine was streaming in through the windows as he made his way to the counselling room. It was at a different time to last week and he didn't have to pass the door to his next lesson. Someone had seen him and shouted out, 'Where you off to, Nick, don't you know where the classroom is, thicko?' Nick hadn't responded. He just kept walking. He suddenly felt very, very alone. In fact he felt sick and a bit light-headed. He hated so much about his life.

He had entered the corridor leading to where the counsellor was. He saw the door ahead; it was open. He knocked, somewhat tentatively, and heard a movement. The counsellor appeared in the doorway. 'Hi, you must be Nick, yeah?'

Nick nodded and although he had glanced up at Simon he now stared ahead of him.

'Come on in and have a seat.'

Nick went in and sat down in one of the chairs. He waited, not sure what was going to happen next.

Simon began speaking. 'So, it's good to see you. I guess it can feel a bit strange.' He had noticed how quiet and withdrawn Nick seemed to be, but that wasn't unusual. Some of the young people he saw were really quiet; others were just in your face the moment they came in, loud and very upfront about things. But his sense already was that this wasn't the kind of young person before him now.

Nick nodded but still didn't say anything. He fidgeted uncomfortably in the seat, still looking ahead and avoiding eye contact.

'There are a few things I need to say. I said them in the assembly, but I do need to repeat them. They are mainly about confidentiality.'

Nick didn't respond.

'Counselling is confidential, and that means that what you say to me stays here, in this room, except in certain cases; for instance, if you tell me that you are a victim of sexual abuse, then while we will discuss it, I will need to pass that on to Mrs Andrews, who is the child protection officer at the school.'

Nick nodded. He remembered that part from the assembly. And it was mentioned in the leaflet that he had been sent after he had referred himself to counselling. But that wasn't his problem though.

'Also, if you are threatening harm to yourself, and I mean serious harm, suicidal thoughts and plans, or maybe cutting yourself severely, then again, I might need to act on that, but we would discuss it and work out what was going to be most helpful for you.'

Nick nodded. There had been times when he had wondered what it would be like to be dead. He hadn't any plans, but he had found himself thinking about it. What would it be like? Nothing? That had its attractions sometimes, but then people talked about going to heaven and stuff, and somehow that sounded really good. But he wondered if it would really be any different.

'So, what brings you along, Nick? Is that OK calling you Nick, or would you prefer something else?'

'Nick's fine.'

'OK, so what's on your mind, Nick?'

> Is this a good opening? It might be too pushy, demanding a response. Another possibility might be 'I'm wondering what has brought you here today', but only if that is what the counsellor is wondering. A crucial feature of person-centred counselling is counsellor authenticity.

Nick went back into silence. He didn't know where to begin and he felt like he was sweating. He felt hot in the room. He took a deep breath and sighed, but said nothing.

Simon noticed the sigh, and wanted to express his sense of how difficult it could be sometimes. He knew how important it was to make a connection with a young person, well, with any client from any age group. Psychological contact, one of the core features of counselling. He recognised that not all young people related well to the formal world of adult counselling, where so often it seemed that there were rules: you sit and you talk, or rather the client sits and talks, and the counsellor listens. But young people sometimes needed more flexibility, more interaction, a clearer sense of the counsellor taking an interest in them.

'Difficult to know what to say? Must seem a bit strange being here. Ever been to counselling before?'

Nick shook his head. He still said nothing.

Simon could feel an increasing desire in himself to reach out to Nick. He sensed his distance, psychological distance, and while he wanted to make a connection, he also acknowledged to himself the need to trust Nick's own process. No doubt he felt a good reason not to say anything. After all, who was he? A stranger. Though something had attracted Nick along. But why should he talk about himself? Maybe he had had experiences in the past that had left him feeling unable to trust people. But he also didn't want the session to simply be silent, which could leave Nick feeling that counselling was pointless and thinking that nothing happened.

'So, how are things at school, at home?'

Nick sat and continued to stare ahead of him. He had lowered his head a little. He just didn't know what to say. He could feel his heart thumping in his chest but he couldn't open his mouth.

'Not easy to talk, yeah?'

Nick nodded though he continued to look downwards.

Simon could accept Nick not saying anything. He was responding, so there was
contact. But he was aware that contact did not need a response. Simply the fact
of his presence was, he sensed, likely to be making an impression on what Nick
was experiencing within his own field of awareness. So Simon maintained the
silence.

Nick was aware of his presence and Simon maintained his feelings of warm acceptance of Nick. Yeah, he felt for him. Couldn't be easy to trust someone you
didn't really know. He respected that Nick would have his reasons for this.
He responded to Nick's nod.

'Yeah, sometimes it's easier to say nothing and simply try to switch it all off.'

If only he could, Nick thought to himself, if only he could. He took another deep
breath.

Simon was so aware of Nick sitting there and how he looked to be struggling.
He had made the effort to be here. He obviously had his reasons. But he,
Simon, didn't want to push him to talk or disclose anything. At the moment
Nick was saying nothing much verbally, but was communicating so much
through choosing to be silent. He couldn't empathise with anything verba-
lised, but he could seek an empathic understanding of Nick's silence. But he
also wanted to avoid too many questions as well. Was Nick wanting to communicate silence, or was it his struggle to speak that was resulting in silence?

'I guess you had things you wanted to say when you first got in touch and
I am wondering how I can help you to maybe talk about them now, if that is
what you still want to do. I'd really like to help you, Nick. I feel that you are
saying so much by sitting there. But there is no rush, take your time, yeah?
Just take it slowly.'

Nick felt a little relieved hearing what the counsellor was saying. Yes, he had
so many things to say, but where to begin? And how would the counsellor
react? And how would he, Nick, feel? He didn't know. It somehow all seemed
very scary. It somehow seemed easier to say nothing, yet that was uncomfortable too.

'I feel really sad. Feel like I'm, I dunno, just don't feel I'm OK.' He was thinking of
the names he was called: 'thicko' was probably the easiest to ignore, but they'd
call him 'the prat' – he really hated that. Bastards, he thought to himself.

'Not feeling OK.' Simon was aware of how intense it was feeling, listening to Nick.
He was talking quite quietly, like he was speaking but lost in his own thoughts
at the same time.

Nick shook his head. 'I just feel so unhappy.'

'It's awful, isn't it, feeling like that?'

Nick nodded, took a deep breath and sighed. 'No one seems to like me.' He lapsed
into silence.

Simon nodded and felt his lips tighten as he did so. Poor kid, he thought, horrible to feel out of everything at his age. He realised his thinking had drifted momentarily to his own childhood. He had had many friends, but there was one lad in his age group, Ian, who nobody liked. He had always been quite an awkward child, and he just got picked on mercilessly. He wondered what had happened to him after he left school. Simon pulled his attention back to Nick, though he wondered whether his thoughts had been drawn to Ian because there was some similarity – as yet undisclosed – between what he had experienced and what Nick was going through. But he wasn't going to start making assumptions.

'Horrible place to be, isn't it, feeling no one likes you.'

'They just keep picking on me, calling me names. I don't know why, they just do and I can't do anything about it.' He could hear the names in his head as he was speaking, 'Nicko the thicko', and 'Hey, prat, come here', and he just felt so awkward, didn't know what to do. Just kept quiet. He hated school, hated it.

'Yeah, kids picking on you, calling you names, not knowing why, and not being able to do anything about it.'

Nick could feel himself instinctively nodding. He so hated it. He could feel his throat getting tight and there were tears in his eyes. He often cried himself to sleep at home, but he tried not to feel this way at school. But somehow, sitting there, somehow he couldn't help himself. He rubbed his eyes and sniffed back the snot that had started to trickle down on to his lip. He got out his handkerchief and blew his nose. The tears continued.

'Sometimes I wish I was dead.'

'That bad, huh?'

Nick nodded. 'I mean, I don't want to be dead, but sometimes I wish I was.'

'Yeah, it's not what you want but sometimes it's so bad . . .'

'They just don't leave me alone. I go to the library at lunch-times just to get away, and I try to keep myself kind of, well, kind of invisible.' He took another deep breath and sighed again. 'Why do they pick on me?'

'That's a question you'd so like answered, yeah, why you?'

Nick nodded. 'I mean, yeah, why me? I fucking hate them all.' As he spoke those last few words he sounded a little different, less resigned to things, a little stronger, like he was finding a voice, a voice that wanted to fight back.

Simon has stayed with his empathy, and with his warmth towards Nick, which will have affected his tone of voice. It has allowed Nick to begin to connect more and more with his experiences and his feeling about them.

'Yeah, you fucking hate them all.' Simon reflected back what Nick had just said.

'I'd like to tell them all to fuck off, I really would. But I can't do it. I just go so quiet. Just want to hide. That's all I do, want to hide.'

Simon nodded. He was aware that throughout Nick had looked down and had been avoiding eye contact. He wanted to convey his warm acceptance of Nick, and he knew that often this was conveyed through his posture and his eye contact, and he felt concerned that maybe this wasn't being received by Nick as he sat there, his eyes all red, looking down at the floor.

'Hide away from it all, hide away.' Simon spoke the words with a certain tone of resignation, seeking to empathise by doing so with his sense of how Nick was feeling about it. He had said how he wanted to tell them to 'fuck off', but he couldn't and did come across as being resigned to it all.

Nick heard Simon speaking, and the way he had spoken. It made him somehow more aware of his wanting to hide away. Yeah, that was the only answer, keep away from the other kids whenever he could, just keep himself to himself. How he hated it.

'I wish they were all dead.'

Simon was struck by the switch from a few minutes ago when Nick was saying he wished he was dead, now wishing the kids who were picking on him, calling him names, were all dead.

Simon stays with his empathy towards Nick's frame of reference. No place for making connections, or highlighting the shift. Nick's not in the place for that. He's only just begun to talk about his feelings. Simon's role is to listen, to let him make visible what he wants to communicate.

'Mhmm, that's what you wish, that they were all dead.'

'Yeah. And I'd kill them, like in the computer games, yeah, take them out, blast them to pieces.'

Simon was aware of a slight anxiety within him as to how much of this was straight fantasy and whether there was actual risk of Nick acting on his wish. But he didn't want to start constraining Nick in saying what he was feeling by questioning him on this. So he continued conveying his empathic understanding of what Nick was saying and experiencing.

'Like in the computer games, blast them to pieces.'

'Yeah, I like playing them, they're really good. Makes me feel good. I am really good at them as well. I spend a lot of time at home playing them.'

'Big part of your life, huh?'

Nick nodded. 'Yeah. I like the ones where there's blood 'n stuff, and when you take someone out they really explode on the screen. Feels for real. Yeah, makes me feel good.'

Simon could see so clearly how all of this might lead Nick into living out in real life something of his fantasy, waste others rather than be picked on, bullied and left feeling awful. In a way, the games were helping Nick to develop or perhaps rather preserve a sense of self that was not afraid to be visible, that was powerful and that felt good. We all needed that, he thought. We all need to feel good. But how experiences in childhood could affect just what we choose in order to get that satisfying feeling. Kids, everywhere, getting a buzz from violent fantasy, maybe compensating for crap experiences in life, though he knew this wasn't always the case, but still, learning that killing, even in fantasy, gave them a buzz, a feeling of pleasure and of achievement. Shit, he thought, what a crazy fucking world we live in.

Simon realised his thoughts had wandered and he knew it was something he needed to clear out in supervision, sound off about probably. He responded to what Nick had been saying. 'Makes you feel good, seeing them explode.'

'Yeah, I love it. Spend hours. Gets me grief, though, kind of never really get enough time for homework. That's always a bit of a rush. Yeah, don't do too good with that, but I don't care. Homework never made me feel good.'

'Never get the same thrill from homework as you do from the computer games, so you end up spending more time on the games, yeah?'

Simon hasn't picked up on the importance to Nick of feeling good.

Nick thought of how often he was in trouble for not doing his homework, having to stay behind after school, but he didn't mind that. Meant he wasn't leaving with everyone else. Less likely to get picked on. 'Yeah. Gets me into trouble but I don't mind.'

'So you really don't mind getting into trouble?' Simon had emphasised the 'really don't mind', wanting to be sure that this really was what Nick was saying and wanting him to hear.

'No, it's good. Stops me getting picked on again. I mean, I live nearby, don't have far to go, but when I leave with everyone else, well, I really have to, you know, kind of keep out of the way. The ones that pick on me, well, they don't all go the way I do, but some do. Sometimes I kind of hang back, other times I try to get away quick.'

'So it really helps getting into trouble and having to stay behind, although sometimes you hang back by choice, other times try to get home fast. Can't leave you looking forward to the journey home, though.'

'No, but I can play the games when I get back, and that's good.'

'That's what you look forward to, yeah, and that's good.'

Nick nodded. 'Yeah. I can kind of forget things. It really helps. But then, well, when I go to bed, I mean, I just start thinking about it and I get sad again.'

'The games only ease things while you're playing them, but they don't take it away.'

Nick nodded his head.

'And you end up feeling sad when you go to bed and try to go to sleep.'

Nick stared ahead of him. Yeah, he thought, night after night. Couldn't stop his brain running, couldn't stop thinking about things. Just felt so sad and worried.

The session continued but Nick didn't say very much. Seemed to be more preoccupied with his own thoughts as Simon looked on. Simon tried to engage with Nick but he seemed determined not to say anything more. After ten minutes or so Simon checked with Nick whether he felt he wanted to continue with the session. In fact, that wasn't what he asked, rather he enquired whether Nick was finding it helpful to be there.

Nick nodded. 'Kind of feel I can relax a bit here although it never really goes away.'

'Mhmm. You can relax but, yeah, it never really goes away.'

Nick sat and somehow felt a little more relaxed. He took a deep breath and let it out with a bit of a sigh, feeling his shoulders drop a bit as he did so.

Simon had noticed the breath and his shoulders dropping. He decided to empathise with the body language.

'Pretty tense, huh, but good to relax a little?'

Nick nodded. It felt good having someone just giving him a bit of time. He never seemed to get that much. The teachers didn't seem to, well, didn't seem to care much. He kind of felt pretty much out of things a lot of the time. He had a few friends, and they'd kind of make time together, but somehow they seemed to have pulled away from him as the name calling had got worse. He just felt more and more alone. He wished it would stop. He wished he could blast them all to bits. Bastards, he thought to himself, fucking bastards.

As the silence continued Simon had noticed that Nick's shoulders had tightened up again. He guessed that whatever Nick was thinking about was making him tense. He didn't want to invade Nick's choice to be silent, but he made a conscious effort of noting the body language, and waited, seeking to maintain his attitude of unconditional positive regard for Nick, who was sitting and looking down at the floor, picking at the hem of his trousers.

Simon, through his empathy for what Nick's body language appeared to be conveying, has offered Nick the opportunity to engage more with his feelings. This he is doing, although he is also preoccupying himself with his trouser hem. The counsellor allows him time and space to be with what is present for him, seeking to offer a safe and supportive environment for him to be with his feelings, a place where he may begin to feel accepted and acceptable.

'I really hate feeling like this, and I hate them all.' Nick closed his eyes and began to cry softly. 'I can't stop them, and I can't tell anyone.'

Simon empathised with what Nick was saying and added the question which was now present for him, 'Is there anyone you want to tell?' He realised that in asking this he was probably going to take Nick away from his feelings, but he had mentioned not being able to tell anyone and it felt important to offer the opportunity to explore this further.

'I can't tell the teachers, I don't think they'd do anything, and if they did, it'd only get worse. So what's the point. My dad's attitude would be to tell me to get on with it, grow up, probably start to teach me to fight them. He has said that in the past, that if I had any trouble he'd show me how to look after myself. But that won't work.'

'So you don't think you can tell the teachers or your father because of the reaction, and it might make it worse, yeah?'

Nick nodded.

Simon was aware that Nick was not the only child who had come to him because of bullying. It seemed that the school wasn't really addressing the problem. Seemed to him that everyone was so stressed with just coping with the demands on them that they didn't have much left to give to worrying about it or doing anything about it. But he didn't want to do anyone an injustice either. Shit, he thought, my mind's wandered off. Yet even as he thought this, he also was aware of wondering whether he should say something to a member of staff about it. He produced reports and made reference to the kind of issues that came up, but they were annually and he was some months away from the next one. The bullying issue certainly seemed to have got worse this autumn term. He didn't know why. He was aware that part of his role was liaison with the pastoral management staff and the teachers, particularly the year tutors.

The fact that the counsellor has become preoccupied with his own thoughts indicates the impact that the bullying issue has had on him. It is a supervision issue. It is likely to also mean that he should take action, draw someone's attention to it, while maintaining client confidentiality if that is the client's wish.

'Can you do anything, I mean, can you say something to someone?'

Simon was aware that he hadn't really been listening, but he had heard what Nick was saying although he knew he had still been in his own thoughts.

'I can. What you say is confidential, and I wouldn't mention you specifically unless that was what you wanted.'

'I just want the teachers to know, you know, that it's a problem and how, you know, how it makes me feel. I mean, not just me, it's happening to others. You must have other kids coming and talking to you.'

Simon nodded. 'Yeah, it does seem to be getting worse and as you were speaking then I was thinking about who needs to be made aware. Nick, how would you feel if I was to say to the pastoral care people and to the headmaster what I am picking up. No names. No reference to you or to anyone specific. Just highlight it as being an issue that needs addressing?'

Nick looked up. 'Would you? I mean ...' Nick lapsed back into silence. It had seemed like such a good idea, but then the thought: what if *they* found out he had talked about it. He looked down again and returned to his labours with the hem of his trousers.

'You seemed momentarily enthusiastic about me telling someone, but then ...' Simon let the sentence trail off as he waited to see if Nick felt able to elaborate on what he had, and was, experiencing.

'I guess I'm worried about what would happen if they find out, you know, the bastards that keep having a go at me.'

Simon nodded. 'Yeah, that's a real concern for you, isn't it, what if they find out.' Simon noted in himself that he wasn't tempted to try to reassure Nick, not at this stage anyway. He felt it important to stay with him, listen to his concerns, let Nick know that he, Simon, was hearing those concerns, and then see how things developed.

The person-centred counsellor is going to want to stay with the client's inner world. Here, the counsellor is aware of what might have been said, but recognises that this is Nick's time and he needs to be trusted to find his own way through what he is experiencing. There is opportunity for Nick to grow and find his own voice, but this could be diminished if the counsellor were to rush in and try and make everything better, or dismiss Nick's concerns, justifying it as being for the greater good. The reality is that Nick is the client, struggling with the pain of being a target for bullying, but he now has someone – Simon – listening to him, taking him seriously, and we cannot be sure what the outcome of this will be in terms of Nick's developing sense of self.

'Be awful. I can't face that, not now, not yet.' He took a deep breath. 'But it is good to have this, to talk.' Nick had a thought. 'I don't suppose you could see me during the lunch-break?'

Simon smiled, he knew what he was thinking – maybe Nick wanted to come at a time so as to avoid the bullying. 'Want to have a bit of space, safe space?'

This isn't exactly empathy because the client hadn't mentioned a safe space, but it is something present within the client's thinking that Simon has picked up on and has voiced. Sometimes a counsellor intuitively knows what is present for the client, or motivating a comment that they make, and it can be valuable and therapeutic to listen to and voice this.

Nick nodded. He felt like he was being understood. 'Yeah, that would be good, you know, really good. Lunch is 12.45 and we start lessons at 2.00pm. I can come straight here after eating, that would be really good. Can I?' Nick was aware of feeling really hopeful and yet kind of anxious in case he was told 'no'. The thought of one lunch-time each week away from it felt so good. 'Can I?'

Simon had got his diary out, and yes, he could. It wasn't going to be a problem. And he could see from the expression on Nick's face just how important it was. Poor kid, he thought. The expression on his face really is telling me how much this name calling is getting to him.

'OK, so I'll be free from 1.00pm next Thursday, OK? You get here as soon as you can.'

'That's great.'

'But it looks like time's nearly up for today, Nick. I'm not going to talk to anyone about the bullying; I really do recognise how difficult that feels for you. So let's put that on hold, just for the moment, yeah? You've really been with some difficult stuff, but I can sense how good it seems for you to know you can come back for appointments on a Thursday lunch-time.'

'Yeah. It's been good. Thanks.' He got up and picked up his bag. As he left the room Nick could feel himself feeling good; he hadn't actually felt that way at school for the longest while. It really did feel good and he wanted more of that feeling. Yeah, he wanted to hang on to this. He'd nearly said it was OK to tell someone, but he didn't. That was too much. As he walked along the corridor he heard someone call out behind him, the usual stuff. He didn't really pay it any attention. Just kept walking to his next lesson. He didn't like it; he could feel himself feeling different, like it was making his good feeling kind of disappear. Fucking bastard, he thought to himself, and muttered quietly under his breath, 'One day, one fucking day, I'll get you.'

Simon was left pondering the session. What was that rhyme, 'Sticks and stones may break my bones, but words will never hurt me.' Bullshit, he thought to himself. Names hurt, and they stick. Emotional wounds don't always heal quite as well as physical ones. They can scar, and the scars can remain for a lifetime. Simon thought about the person-centred theory around introjects and conditions of worth. His jaw tightened and he wondered at how so many kids came through it all. And how many end up in therapy as adults, or become therapists themselves.

The term 'conditions of worth' applies to the conditioning that is frequently present in childhood, and at other times in life, when a person experiences that their sense of worth is conditional on their doing something, or behaving, in a certain way. The person feels they have to be a certain way to have self-worth. With this come attendant beliefs that there are certain ways that they should not be, as this will negate any sense of self-worth. The person is left experiencing a need to behave in certain ways in order to achieve a sense of self-worth.

'Introjects' are beliefs that the person has about themselves. They have been described in person-centred theory as 'an evaluation taken in from the outside and symbolised as defining a dimension of the Self' (Mearns and Thorne, 2000, p. 108). The person seeks to live according to these introjects – for instance, beliefs such as: I am successful, I am a perfectionist, I am useless, I am unlovable, I feel warmth for everyone. But they are difficult to live up to, often offering extremes, and because they are taken in from outside, they are not genuine aspects of the person. People may carry conflicting introjects, leaving them doomed to fail at one whenever they achieve the other.

Points for discussion

- How would you have responded to a young person not attending their first session?
- Evaluate Simon's handling of the silences. How might you have responded differently?
- If you were Nick, do you think you would you have felt supported during that session and why?
- At what point might you decide to communicate an issue such as verbal bullying to teaching staff?
- Were there any crucial moments in the session for the developing relationship between Nick and Simon and, if there were, what were they?
- Consider the 'conditions of worth' and 'introjects' that might have surfaced for you had you been counselling Nick in this session.
- Write your own notes for the session as if you were the counsellor.

CHAPTER 13

Supervision 1

'I want to spend the last 20 minutes talking about a new client, a young lad at the school, who I saw for the first time last Thursday.' Simon always wanted to at least check in with new clients as soon as possible in supervision, to first of all keep his supervisor up to date on who he was seeing, but also to use it as an opportunity to pick up anything related to how he was reacting to the client and the impact it could be having on the quality of the therapy he was offering. Often he didn't feel he had anything specific to raise, but that wasn't the case with Nick.

'OK, so, what do you want to tell me?' Sarida left it open for Simon to speak as he felt he wanted to. She trusted him to know if he had something he needed to say. He came across to her as so sensitive to the kids he worked with – not just as a counsellor, he also occasionally spoke about his own children. He just seemed so cut out for working with them somehow, had that touch that you can't learn in books, and probably not learn on training courses either. It seemed to her that with some people what they needed most from counselling training was an opportunity to enhance their self-awareness, do work on themselves so that they could be authentic and congruently aware. She momentarily thought back to her own training and all the encounter groups that had helped her so much in coming to know herself. It had been tough, being Asian and Muslim. She had been the only non-white on the course, but she'd stuck it out and it had really helped.

People like Simon were natural listeners and seemed able to relate to people as easily as breathing. He seemed to have boundless warmth for the kids he worked with as well. And she knew that if he had something to say, if something hadn't felt right in the sessions, he would be keen to get a handle on it.

Simon began by describing Nick and then moved on to the issue and its impact on him. 'It's bullying, verbal, he's getting a lot of it, poor kid, and he doesn't know what to do.' Nick shook his head. 'But what he is doing is using computer games to kind of release his pent-up feelings – at least, that's how it's coming across. You know, those games where you're killing people all over the place – bloody scary things for kids to get addicted to, but anyway, that's another rant for later. He's using them and imagining he's blasting the bullies. In a way, it kind of feels like a healthy psychological process in that it is at least helping him to release, but it's also getting him into a particularly murderous frame of mind.' Sarida was aware of how fast Simon was talking. 'Really fires you up, yes?'

Empathic responses are not always directed by the content of what is said; the tone of what is said is also a key aspect of what is communicated. The supervisor identifies this, offering an opportunity to explore this further.

'Too right, and I know it's getting to me. I've seen a few kids this term with differ-ent kinds of bullying problems, but this one has got to me, and I know it's partly the computer games thing. Nick seems a bit of a loner, you know; most of the others I've seen seem to have close friends and family they've talked to. But Nick doesn't.'

'So the other kids have talked to their parents but not Nick, and the computer games are leaving you feeling ...?' Sarida left the sentence open, not sure quite how it was leaving Simon feeling.

'I feel for him, and I feel for the fact of what he is having to do to cope, which I don't think is healthy, but I guess it's helping him or he wouldn't be doing it, you know?' Simon was aware of feeling unsettled in himself, and he voiced this. 'It leaves me feeling unsettled.'

'Unsettled?' Sarida was wondering what Simon was meaning and in the back of her mind was what impact it would be having on the quality of his empathy for Nick.

A very brief response yet one that captures the primary feeling that is present for the supervisee, again offering the opportunity for the supervisee to con-nect more fully with what is present for them and to explore their experience.

'Yeah, kind of uneasy. That sort of churning kind of sense in my stomach. I mean, part of me feels that at least Nick is coming and he seems to be engaging. Oh yes, and he was suddenly visibly brighter when we arranged for future sessions to be during his lunch-break – giving him a break from the verbal bullying. Yes, I'd forgotten that. He really changed, he was suddenly so different and while I kind of acknowledged it, it was right at the end of the session. He must have been so aware of how it felt and I just wonder how long that lasted, and how he was then left feeling once the verbal started again, you know? I mean, he could feel a little more resilient, but he might find the contrast really difficult to handle.'

Sarida nodded. She was quite calm by nature and she was very conscious of how Simon was presenting. She wouldn't go so far as to say agitated, but he was animated. She wasn't feeling that way at all. She felt for Nick. She knew what bullying could be like as well. She had had a tough time at school as a Muslim. All kinds of names. She'd not been hit, but she'd been spat at and she had spoken about it at home but had not got any sympathy. Rather it was explained to her that it was something to be proud of, and that she should take the abuse for the glory of her religion. Looking back now she didn't agree. It was abuse and steps should have been taken. But that was then. She was very different now. She had moved on, though she knew that she still carried sensitivities from those times.

'I was just being aware of my own experience, but also wanted to acknowledge my sense of your animation. There is something about Nick that has really touched you, Simon, and I am wondering what impact that is having on your empathy, your congruence, and whether your positive regard might be at risk of being conditional in some way.'

'I'm also aware that I drifted away from him a few times as well, caught in my own thoughts. On one occasion thinking about someone I remembered from school who was bullied. It's a real theme at that school. I did mention to Nick, no, he suggested it, although I was thinking about it, about maybe mentioning it to someone. He was at first momentarily quite enthusiastic, but then he lapsed back into silence and said he was concerned what would happen if the ones who were bullying him found out that he had talked about it. So I said I wouldn't say anything at this stage. He seemed OK with that.'

'So he seemed OK with you not mentioning it. And what about you?'

'Me?'

'Mhmm. How do you feel having agreed not to mention it to anyone at the school.'

Supervision can become very client-centred in the sense of talking about the client; however, the supervisor is also concerned about the impact of the therapeutic relationship on the supervisee. The supervisee is enabled to understand themselves and their reactions more clearly, uncovering areas of unrecognised incongruence that might impact on the quality of their empathy. The result is a counsellor who can be more fully and clearly present with their client, able to respond accurately to what is being said with the minimum of interference from material within their own experience that is irrelevant to the client's inner world.

Shit, thought Simon, I hadn't really thought about that. He was suddenly aware that that uneasy feeling had returned and his arms felt a funny kind of tingling sensation. 'Uneasy. That feeling again.' He stopped and thought about it. What was he feeling? Where was he feeling it?

'Mhmm. That uneasy feeling again. Makes you feel uneasy knowing you've agreed not to say anything.'

He nodded slowly, looking into Sarida's eyes as he did so. He swallowed. 'It feels a heavy uneasiness, like it's heavy in my stomach.'

'Heavy like you feel full?'

'No. Just heavy, but moving, churning, like something soft and heavy just churning around inside me.'

'Soft and heavy, churning around inside you.' Sarida kept her response simple
and focused to allow Simon to connect more deeply with what he had just conveyed to her.
Simon took a deep breath and let the air out slowly. Ian came back into his mind
again, the kid from his school who was bullied. He could see him clearly, standing there on the school playing fields, being laughed at and jeered by the other
kids. He was with them, but he wasn't joining in. God, it was clear in his mind.
He hadn't thought about that incident in years. He could remember walking
away, walking away, having to get away.
Sarida sat with the silence that had arisen, maintaining her focus on Simon and
awaiting whatever he felt he wanted to say. She commented, 'You look suddenly
a long way away', which was how he felt to her, somehow strangely distant.

Sarida is responding to her experience of Simon as he sits looking distant –
again, not a focus on what is being said but more on his way of being.

Simon nodded. He had heard Sarida but he didn't feel any great motivation to
respond. He was somehow held by that past experience. It wasn't that he was
remembering anything else, rather he had stopped remembering anything; he
just felt stuck, somehow, powerless to move on. He was suddenly aware that
his eyes were watering and he looked up, taking another deep breath.
'I was reliving an incident at school. The lad, Ian, was verbally taunted. I can
see it happening and I remember walking away. I hadn't joined in, but I was
with those who were doing the jeering. But I left. I just couldn't stay.' He tightened his lips. 'As I'm speaking now I've just flashed back to one moment,
before I walked away. He caught my eye. I walked away, Sarida, I walked away.
I couldn't do anything. I felt utterly powerless.' He shook his head. 'I couldn't . . .
oh shit . . .'
'You couldn't . . . ?' Sarida responded, speaking softly, not wanting to disturb
Simon from what he was reliving. He was clearly connecting with some powerful feelings that he hadn't perhaps engaged with for a while. Certainly he had
not talked this way before in relation to other clients at the school.
Simon shook his head and smiled, although it was a weak smile. 'I was about to
say that "I couldn't stomach it". Yeah, I couldn't and at some level I still can't.
The not being able to do anything. It's a big part of my motivation in what I do.
And I know it but somehow it has become very real for me today.'
'Nick's helplessness has touched into your helplessness?' Sarida regarded her
response as one of informed speculation.

Sarida has got a little ahead of Simon here, making a connection for him
that perhaps would have been more valuable for him had he made the connection from the focus of his experience of helplessness. However, Simon
can acknowledge this and continues to explore his experience.

Simon nodded. 'Yeah. That's what's got to me. And I know it's about the question of "Will counselling be enough?" Should I do more? And part of me wants to do more. Part of me! It's a damn big part of me wanting to do more. Yet I also want to help Nick find his own voice, his own strength as well. I really want for that to happen.'

'Really want Nick to find his own voice, his own strength. That's a real goal for you, yes?'

Simon agreed. 'Yes, my goal, my goal. Shit. What a mess. I mean, there's me wanting to do more, wanting to do something to make a difference, a real practical difference with crap he's having to put up with. And there's this other part that has goals for him. I'm person-centred. I don't have goals.'

'Really?' Sarida knew she was playing devil's advocate. She knew that counsellors have goals, whatever their theoretical base. Even achieving psychological contact with a client is a goal.

'Yeah, I know. I think he's hooked that helplessness. I'm left realising how much that may be part of my motivation in this work. I mean, I kind of knew it but it's like I sort of know it even more now, and need to watch it because it will affect, does affect, no, has affected how I am. I can't push. I have to accept Nick where he is, and I have to carry that tension in me of wanting to alert the school but also wanting to maintain a confidential space for Nick. He made it clear he didn't want me to say anything and I feel I must respect that. He may change his mind and I hope he does, and I've got to be sure I don't encourage this. I really have to watch that.' Simon glanced at the clock. 'Time's getting on. And I haven't had a chance for my rant at computer games. Oh well, another time maybe.'

'I want to acknowledge that it seems that rant would be important for you, but I also want to check out where you are now given what we have talked about.'

'I need to really be there for and with Nick. I'm sensitive to the helplessness of my own past powerlessness and I mustn't try compensating for that in my work with Nick. He has to travel at his pace. I have to give him my attention and offer him a supportive relationship and help him, well, help him with whatever he needs to do to come through this with some degree of psychological health. And as I say that the thought of him spending hours on a computer fantasising about blasting the bullies to kingdom come doesn't feel healthy at all. But I have to hold that; it's my stuff. He's doing what he needs to do at this time and maybe if I can give him quality time and attention he may need less of that and begin to explore other ways of coping or dealing with the situation. I hope so. But I must accept him and not try and change him to fit my prejudices.'

The supervision session drew to an end. Simon felt much clearer in himself as he left, although he was also aware of the effects of the intensity of the session. He felt sharper and drained at the same time. He took it steadily as he drove home, aware that he was lost in thought and having to make the effort to concentrate. Yes, he thought, Nick needs some space, his space, and he doesn't need it full of my attitudes and compensations for my past experiences. He felt determined to offer Nick a quality therapeutic relationship and allow him to decide his focus and the pace. Yeah, he somehow felt he had reconnected with the attitudinal values and principles of person-centred working, and that felt good. He felt more positive. The uneasy feeling had passed. Yes, he thought, I'm going to help Nick find his way through all this.

Points for discussion

- How would you describe the tone and nature of the supervisory relationship between Sarida and Simon?
- Did Simon bring all the issues that needed to be explored to this session?
- Contrast this session with supervision as you have experienced it.
- If you had to choose a word or words other than 'supervision' to describe this process, what would you use?

CHAPTER 14

Counselling session 3: the need to alert the school to bullying

Nick arrived for his next session a few minutes late.

'Sorry 'bout that, the dinner queue wasn't too quick, happens sometimes.'

'Yeah, can't do much about that.' Simon paused, then continued, 'So, how do you want to use today's session?'

'Don't know really. Felt good leaving here last week but it kind of faded as the week went on. Felt able to ignore people after I left here, that I had something to kind of look forward to, a place to get a break from it at least once a week. And that felt good.'

'Felt good knowing you were going to have at least one lunch-time free of the verbal, yeah?'

Nick nodded. 'But it still goes on, you know, and actually I've thought of a way of getting a break from it another day. I'm going to join a music club. Not sure what it's about, but there was a note up on a notice board, for Wednesday lunch-times, which is great 'cos it will give me two days free of grief, and somehow it makes it all a little easier. I hadn't really thought of doing anything like that before, but having realised I could have the counselling on a Thursday lunch-time, and knowing how different I was feeling, well, I thought, yeah, let's give it a go. So it starts next week and I'm looking forward to it.'

'So, you were feeling different once you knew you could have counselling on a Thursday lunch-time and that opened up other possibilities.'

Nick nodded. 'Yeah. But it's still going on.' He looked down as he said it. Somehow, to Simon, Nick seemed to be ashamed that he wasn't able to stop it, but that was very much his own speculation and he didn't voice it. Rather he stayed with what Nick had conveyed to him verbally.

'Still going on.'

Nick didn't respond. He was feeling helpless. He knew that whatever he did, it wasn't going to stop it happening. Even if he did things every lunch-time there were still other times when he knew he'd get picked on. It just didn't seem fair.

'Not easy to talk about, huh?' Simon wanted to acknowledge the difficulty he sensed that Nick was having. As soon as he said it he realised how much he had made an assumption. It might be the difficulty in talking about it that was causing the silence; maybe Nick simply didn't want to talk about it. Simon decided to keep quiet and let Nick say what he needed to say, and if he needed to maintain silence then he would respect that.

A client in silence has not stopped communicating. They may be simply wanting to be silent, to be with their own thoughts and feelings. Being respectful of that need can be important. However, checking out whether the client wishes to be in silence, or whether they require help in exploring and communicating whatever is present for them can sometimes be valuable.

Nick heard Simon. No, it wasn't easy to talk about it. He had felt really positive last week, but that had faded as the taunting had continued. Bastards, he thought, fucking bastards. I hate them, I want to waste them. As the thoughts passed through his mind he felt himself tense. His hands were clenched and his jaw was tight. He wished he had a gun, a ray gun like the one in the new game he'd got at the weekend. Then he'd show them. Then he'd make them notice him.

Time passed and Nick remained silent, although to Simon it didn't somehow seem awkward, at least not after the first minute. Nick simply looked lost in his thoughts. He wondered about saying anything but he was mindful of not wanting to interrupt whatever process was occurring for Nick. Finally he said, 'If you want to say anything I'm hear to listen, Nick.' He spoke softly, and waited.

Nick heard Simon speak but it seemed distant. He ignored it, he was feeling good now, yeah, he could see himself wasting them, every fucking one of them. He smiled to himself. He felt strong. They could call him names, and yes, he hated it, but he knew that one day, one day, he'd get back at them. Yeah, he'd get them. He hadn't realised that his facial expression had changed to a kind of sneer. Simon had noticed it though, and found himself wondering what Nick must be thinking about. But he still wanted to respect Nick's right to silence.

A few more minutes passed. Simon felt an increasing urge to say something. He couldn't rationalise it, but it had become more present. He felt that while clearly Nick was thinking about something, it had somehow made him feel distant, and he wanted to regain psychological contact with him, or at least remind Nick again of his presence.

'Seems like you have a lot going on for you, Nick, and I'm wondering if you want to tell me about it.'

'I'll get them, you know, one day, I'll get them.'

He sounded very strong and somehow there was a note of real malice in his voice.

'One day, huh, one day you'll get them, yeah? You sound pretty sure of yourself.'

'I am. They may have the better of me now, but one day . . .'

'Mhmm. Got some plans, yeah?'

Nick felt a sensation of unease. Yeah, he'd got plans, but he didn't want to talk about them. They were his, and for him to know, nobody else. Couldn't trust anyone else. No. He'd stay quiet and wait. 'Yeah, I'll get back at them somehow, sometime.'

Simon nodded. 'You sound pretty determined.'

'I am. They've made my life a misery. Maybe when I get older, maybe I'll grow bigger than them and then I can beat the shit out of them. That's what I want to do. But not yet. I'll keep out of their way.'

'That's what you want to do some day, beat the shit out of them, but not yet.'

Hearing that being said sounded good, Nick thought as he sat. He was still looking down, not wanting to catch Simon's eyes. Yeah, one day. He'd blast them. His mind drifted back to the game. He was really good at it now. Getting invincible. That's how he wanted to be, so no one would ever mess with him.

The concept of himself as being invincible, generated through the games, is a kind of reaction against the feelings of helplessness that occur in his daily life at school. It is a kind of reactive compensation, a way for his structure of self to cope with the overwhelming feelings of helplessness. It is an important part of Nick's structure of self, a kind 'compensatory introject' to enable him to create a hopeful future and a sense of personal power.

Nick took a deep breath, and sighed. Somehow the ideas in his head suddenly felt small. He felt small. He remembered how they had been taunting him before school. He'd been dropped off early. He hadn't wanted to be, but his mum was going out and wanted to drop him off at school early. He had pleaded with her not to do that, but let him leave the house himself a bit later. But she wouldn't have anything of it. Yet he couldn't bring himself to say why. He didn't think she'd understand. She was always so busy, never seemed to have time for him. Even when she wasn't doing anything much, like watching TV, she didn't want to be interrupted. It was one of the reasons he spent so much time in his room. It was so boring being downstairs. He suddenly felt very alone and the sense of helplessness spread back over him once more.

Simon had sensed a change, though he couldn't quite get a fix on it. But Nick looked different. He somehow seemed to have returned to being a small boy again. It wasn't that he had thought that he had become something else, but somehow he seemed smaller now, and he had that anxious look back on his face that he had noticed from time to time.

'You look worried again.'

Simon communicates his empathic sense of what is present for Nick through the expression he sees on his face. He wants to let Nick know that he is registering something of what is present for Nick, offering opportunity for further dialogue.

Nick nodded. 'Yeah, for a while I was feeling strong but then, well, the feeling of what's the point, I mean, what's the point. I can never win. It was horrible this morning. Three of them just kept having a go. They kept me cornered. I knew something like that would happen. I didn't want to come to school early, but she made me come. I hate her for that.'

Simon guessed Nick was talking about his mother, but he didn't check it out. Rather he stayed with the feelings. 'You really hate her for making you come to school early.' He spoke the words with a little bit more energy and volume.

Nick clenched his fists again. He could feel a surge of anger and he tightened his fists further and his chest. He just held them in front of him. He just felt so angry, so full of rage. It was like his whole body was bursting with it. He eventually slammed his fists down on the arms of the chair. 'I fucking hate her.' He shouted the words out uncontrollably. Then burst into tears.

Simon handed him a tissue. He didn't say anything. He let the tears continue to flow for a while. Nick was sniffing now and blew his nose on the tissue. Simon handed him another. 'I-I don't really hate her, not really . . . but I do as well. I was really scared this morning. Thought they'd never stop.'

'Yeah, mixed feeling, part of you hates her, part of you doesn't, but it was really scary this morning, feeling they weren't going to stop.' Simon felt sure the concern he was feeling would be visible on his face.

A powerful empathic acknowledgement of what Nick is feeling. The presence of his concern as well will also have created a sense of Simon's genuineness in his warmth for Nick.

Nick nodded and glanced up at Simon, noticing how he looked concerned. That felt strangely reassuring, although it didn't change anything. His eyes were uncomfortable and he rubbed them. They were now very red, and his cheeks were quite blotchy. 'I don't think I can take much more, not like this morning. I don't know what to do. I want it to stop but I can't stop it. I can't. I don't know what to do.'

'Yeah, you can't stop it, you don't know what to do, they just keep on and on, yeah?' Simon could feel his heart going out to Nick. That response had been empathic to Nick's words but not to desperation. He added, 'What do you want to do?'

'I want someone to stop it.' Nick sat and thought about it. He wanted Simon to stop it. 'Can you do something?'

'What would you like me to do?'

'Talk to someone about it.'

'I can talk to Mr Davies, the pastoral care facilitator. I don't have to mention your name.'

'Don't mention my name, but I just want it to stop.' Nick had looked up again now, and his eyes seemed to be so round and pleading. Simon could feel himself taking a deep breath.

'OK, but let's decide together what I should say. How does that seem?'

Simon wanted Nick to feel part of this process, to realise that he had a voice, that even if he couldn't bring himself to say things directly, what he wanted to say would be passed on and taken seriously. Simon is attempting to help Nick develop a sense that he does have power to be heard and to make a difference. He wants to empower Nick while being sensitive to Nick feeling that he needs someone else to say something.

Nick nodded. 'I want the teachers to be aware and to try and do something.'

'What do you think would help?' Simon sought to encourage Nick to come up with his own ideas, hoping that if he could then convey these to the head of pastoral care then maybe they might happen, and Nick would benefit from witnessing this.

'It isn't just me. No one seems to bother. You don't see teachers much at break-times.'

'So the teachers aren't around and the verbal bullying is happening to lots of kids?'

'Yeah. I mean, I don't know, just make them aware. They just piss off to their room and don't seem bothered what happens.'

Simon nodded. 'So it seems to you that they don't care. And you want them to care?'

'Yeah. I want it brought out into the open.'

Simon was still nodding. 'Out in the open. How would you like that to happen?'

'I'd like it to be made a theme, perhaps at assembly, yeah, that would be good. Someone to talk about it at assembly, and really, you know, frighten the bastards. Yeah, really make it clear – zero tolerance, we had that in a lesson the other day. Well, we need fucking zero tolerance here.'

Simon was aware that he agreed with Nick and felt he wanted to convey that to him. He thought that in doing this he was not only being authentic, he was also helping Nick to realise that he had ideas that adults could take seriously. 'I think you're right, Nick. It has no place in schools. It doesn't have a place anywhere, but let's start here, yeah?'

Nick nodded. He suddenly felt a little more hopeful again, a sense that maybe something might happen. Simon seemed genuinely concerned and he, Nick, felt that Simon was taking him seriously. That felt good. Yeah. He liked the idea that maybe he could make something happen to change things.

Simon had noticed the expression on Nick's face change. 'Feels good, doesn't it, when you begin to believe you can maybe make a difference?'

Nick nodded again, a little more vigorously this time.

'So what do you want the teachers to hear? What would you want to tell them?'

Nick thought for a moment. 'I'd want to tell them to stop the bullies, make them back off. I mean, really make it difficult for them. They're messing my head up, they mess lots of us up. Bastards.'

'Mhmm. What else?' Simon wanted to encourage Nick to really express what he wanted to see happen. At the moment he was still firing off his feelings.

'Well, I think the whole school needs to talk about it – assembly. That's where it needs to be.'

Simon was aware that he had an open invitation to speak at the assembly. He had done recently but maybe this issue needed addressing, and perhaps he could be part of that.

'So, have it addressed at assembly, so the whole school is involved.'

'Yeah, maybe we can make it a school project.' Nick's mind was beginning to run a little faster now. 'Posters on the walls. We could do them, everyone could do them, saying how bullying is wrong. We could do that in art lessons. That would be good. And make the bullies realise what it feels like to be picked on all the time.'

'OK, so some kind of school project involving posters and getting the bullies to realise what it feels like to be picked on all the time, yeah?'

Nick was really getting into it now. 'And what about some kind of school play, or something, yeah, that would be really good too.'

'Mhmm, school play, something to involve the whole school.'

Nick nodded, but then his manner changed. 'But then, well, it probably won't happen. I mean, seems a great idea sitting here, but it won't happen. Teachers have other things to do. It'll still go on.' He looked down and began to pick at his trousers.

Nick is unable as yet to sustain his optimistic feelings. The part of himself that is carrying them is newly forming and is still easily overwhelmed by the part of himself that knows it is pointless. Both are aspects of Nick's nature, and each needs to be acknowledged and accepted by the counsellor. The counsellor could try to bolster up the optimism, thinking it would be helpful, make the client feel better. But, in fact, it would leave the client with perhaps a false hope introduced from outside. The client's reality needs to be empathically understood by the counsellor. The person-centred counsellor will want to honour all that is present for and within their client, trusting that the actualising tendency will take the client towards a fuller engagement with those aspects of their nature that they find most satisfying. The therapeutic relationship can offer the supportive climate in which the client can not only dare face the hopelessness but also begin to tentatively embrace the optimistic.

'That's what you feel, it probably won't happen, the teachers are too busy, what's the point.'

Yes, thought Nick, what's the point. He felt stuck inside himself, suddenly tired of it all and just didn't know what more to say. He continued to sit, picking at his trousers, not looking up.

Simon was aware of the profound shift in mood and how the enthusiasm that had seemed one moment so present had seemingly evaporated into hopelessness. He remained silent, holding his attention on Nick. He fleetingly felt an urge to offer to do something, but knew that was a rescue. His focus must be on Nick and allowing his own process to flow within the experience of the therapeutic alliance.

Nick felt lost in himself as he sat there. He wasn't thinking in those terms; he wasn't really thinking at all. Rather he just felt very sad. He just felt it was all so hopeless. So he came to counselling once a week and there was that club, the music club, he was going to go to. But it didn't stop him feeling bad. In fact, he felt bad most of the time. It was always on his mind. Never got a break from it except when he was asleep, but he didn't sleep too well. Found his head wouldn't switch off in the evening.

Simon could feel his heart going out to Nick, who looked so miserable sitting there. Simon empathised with the last thing Nick had said as it felt as though it was still very much present. 'It'll still go on . . .'

'Can't really get away from it. Can't stop thinking about it, worrying about it.' He paused before continuing, and as he did so he looked up. 'Why do they do it? Am I so awful, so different?'

'It really leaves you questioning yourself.'

'I feel so useless sometimes, so pissed off with everything, and so tired. And I'm not really concentrating much in classes, keep drifting off. The teachers – some of them – have noticed, and it's got me into trouble a couple of times.'

'Useless, pissed off and tired, huh?' Simon had intended to empathise with the rest of what Nick had said but he didn't get a chance.

Nick was breathing deeply and sighing. 'And it makes me, I don't know . . . I just don't know.'

Simon could feel himself wanting to reassure Nick in some way. Poor kid, he thought, the bastards just don't know what they're doing to him. Or maybe they do, and get a kick out of it. He realised his mind was made up. He was going to do something about the bullying. It was likely not only Nick was being affected this badly. It wasn't on.

'Nick, I really want to say that I hear the struggle you're having and it seems to me that it has got out of hand, affecting your sleep, your schoolwork, getting you into trouble. It's unacceptable. I want to do something.' As he said those last words he immediately wondered if he had gone too far, but the reaction from Nick was immediate. He burst into tears. Simon passed him a tissue. The tears continued.

'I'm not going to say "it's OK" because it's plainly not OK, Nick. You've had enough of it, yeah?'

Nick nodded through the tears. Sniffing, he rubbed his eyes and put his head in his hands, and nodded as he did so.

'OK. Here, have another tissue. Do you want a glass of water or something?'

Nick nodded again. Simon was fortunate in that the room had a sink and there were some plastic cups. He ran the cold tap for a few moments, filled the cup and returned to where Nick was sitting. He was still rubbing his eyes. Simon handed him the cup. 'Here you are, Nick.'

Nick took it and drank it in gulps.

'I'm sorry.'

'Sorry?'

'About crying.'

'You needed to cry. It's OK to cry when you need to cry. You're facing up to and struggling to cope with some horrible things.'

Nick nodded. 'I do want it to stop, and I do want something done. It's scary though . . . What will happen?'

Nick being allowed to engage more fully with his feeling of hopelessness and helplessness has brought him to a point at which, when Simon expresses his feelings that in effect enough is enough and he wants to do something, the tension that has built up in Nick is released. As a result he begins again to engage with his sense of wanting something to be done.

'What do you want to happen?'

'I want it to stop. I want the teachers to know that it's happening.'

'To know that it's happening to you, or it's happening generally?'

Nick thought for a moment. 'Both.'

'Sure about that?'

Nick was nodding and looking straight back at Simon. 'Yes.'

'So do you want me to talk to someone in the school about it – I think I really need to go to the headmaster. What do you think? Who do you want to know?'

Nick took a deep breath. That sounded scary. He suddenly could feel himself hesitating. 'I-I'm not sure.'

'OK, maybe that sounds like too big a step, yeah, you're not sure, but you want the teachers to know it is happening?'

Nick nodded but stayed silent.

'I can talk to the pastoral care manager. But he may decide to take it to the headmaster. I think it will end up with him eventually, particularly as this is something that is widespread.'

'Will my name be mentioned?'

'Do you want that? I really want to respect your right to confidentiality, Nick.'

'Yes, but . . .'

'But?'

'Can you just say that it's a problem, but don't mention my name, not yet.' He paused. 'But then, will anything be done?'

'I hope so, Nick. Who would you feel OK with knowing about it?'

Nick thought. He wasn't sure. 'I guess my form teacher, Mrs Abbott.'

'I agree, Nick, I think she needs to know, particularly as it is affecting your work. She needs to know, to understand why you are struggling with your attention.' Simon paused for a moment. 'Do you want to be there as well, and maybe say something?'

Nick hadn't thought of that and he was suddenly aware that he was nodding.

'You're sure?'

'Yes.'

'OK. When? Maybe arrange for her to come next week at the beginning of this time we have. Would that be OK?'

Somehow that felt better. Or would it? A whole week. He'd worry about it, he knew he would. 'Can we do it now?'

'Sure that's what you want?'

Nick nodded.

'I can call the staff room from here. She might not be there, though.'

'Can you try?'

Simon nodded and went over to the phone. Yes, Mrs Abbott was there, and yes, she could come down. Simon said it was a bullying issue and that he had one of her pupils with him who wanted her to be aware.

'She's coming down now. She hasn't got much time because classes begin soon.'

'OK. But I don't know what to say.'

'What do you want her to hear?'

'That there's a lot of bullying going on and that I'm getting called names and that I can't help worrying about it and I . . .'

There was a knock on the door.

'Mrs Abbott,' Simon called out.

'Yes.'

Simon looked back at Nick. 'OK?'

Nick nodded.

'Please come in.'

The door opened and Mrs Abbott, Nick's form teacher, came in. 'Sorry, I've only a few minutes before the next classes. Hello Nick.' She noticed his red eyes. 'What's happened?'

'Nick?' Simon looked at him, inviting him to speak.

Nick looked down again. Suddenly it felt like he didn't want to say anything. His tongue suddenly felt too big for his mouth and he had gone strangely dry. He swallowed. 'I-er, I . . .' He lapsed into silence.

'It's not easy for him to talk about it, Mrs Abbott, but I know he wants to.'

She had turned to Simon as he spoke, but now she looked back to Nick. 'It's not easy to talk about things, Nick, and some things are really hard to talk about. Can you tell me? I'd really like to hear.'

Simon felt relieved that Nick's form teacher had responded in the way that she had. She might have been dismissive, or started looking at her watch and stuff like that, but she didn't. She gave him time to find his words.

'Well, Mrs Abbott, I'm getting called names, all the time, and I'm not the only one. Some people it's worse.' Nick could feel a surge of energy as he spoke, like he had suddenly found his voice and needed to keep talking.

Looks like nervous energy has taken over, Simon thought, as Nick's words began to accelerate.

'Every break, and lunch-times, and in the classroom. They get at me, calling me names like "Nicko the thicko" and stuff, and it's getting to me. They hide my stuff and push me in the corridors and stuff. Not sleeping well, feeling tired. I hate it. And I don't know what to do. But it isn't just me, and I don't want anyone to know that I'm talking to you 'cos it'll make it worse.'

Mrs Abbott replied, telling Nick that she understood, but that it did need to be dealt with. She asked him who was doing it, but Nick wouldn't, no, couldn't say.

She didn't push him after asking him again that he was sure he couldn't tell her. 'So when does it happen, breaks and lunch-times?'

Nick nodded. 'And before school, and sometimes after, and . . . and . . .'

'OK, let me listen out for it happening and I'll intervene, then it won't seem like you've told anyone. How about that?'

Nick nodded.

'And you say there's a lot of bullying going on?'

Nick nodded again.

'I need to discuss this with other teachers. Do your parents know?'

Simon could feel that Nick was getting uncomfortable. He certainly was. Mrs Abbott was taking over and he felt concerned that Nick was struggling.

Simon interjected. 'I don't think they do. It's difficult to tell them, yeah?'

Mrs Abbott thought for a moment. 'I think they need to know.'

'Can you tell them Nick?' Simon intervened, wanting to help Nick feel he had some power in the situation.

Before Nick had a chance to reply, Mrs Abbott responded, 'I think it is OK Nick telling them if he wants to, but I think it has to come from the school as well. But not until I've heard it for myself.' She turned back to Nick. 'But we can talk about that, Nick.' Mrs Abbott turned to Simon. 'Look, I do need to head off to my class now. Nick, what class have you got next?'

'French.'

'OK, do you need a bit more time here?'

Nick nodded.

Simon spoke, 'Yes, we need to end the session.'

'OK, I'll let Mr Stevens know you'll be a few minutes late as I'll be passing his classroom.'

'Thanks, Mrs Abbott.'

She left. Simon looked across to Nick as she closed the door.

'That wasn't easy for you. Well done. How are you feeling?'

'Wobbly. I need to tell Mum and Dad. I'll try talking to Mum first.'

Simon nodded. 'You feel up to that, feel it is what you want to do?'

'I want them to hear it from me first. Not from a letter or a phone call from school.' He paused. 'Don't know what to say, though.'

Simon was aware that he had to end the session soon as well. It was overrunning and eating into the time he had between sessions. But he wanted to help Nick think about what he would say before the session ended.

'We've only got a few minutes left. What would you like them to know?'

Nick thought about it. 'How sad I am, and worried, and how it's affecting me.'

Simon nodded. 'I'm sure they'll want to be there for you, Nick. It's just such a difficult thing to talk about.'

Nick sighed. Yes, he thought, it is. He still didn't know what he'd say. He'd think of something, though. He looked at the clock. His lesson had started. He hated going in when everyone was already there. But he knew he had to.

'Same time next week?'

'Sure. And we'll talk about it again, yeah, and see how the week has gone?'

Nick got up and left. He was very thoughtful. He didn't know what to say to his parents. It sort of felt good that Mrs Abbott knew now; it hadn't been as bad as he had thought it would be. He felt that his name wasn't going to be mentioned. He didn't want anyone finding out it was him. He walked slowly up the stairs; his heart was pounding more as he approached the classroom door. Oh shit, he thought, he hadn't got his lesson books. In the rush for lunch and getting to the session he'd forgotten. He panicked and turned away and went back to his form room. He knew Mrs Abbott was there and she wouldn't mind him getting his books – at least, he hoped she wouldn't. He felt more comfortable doing that than going straight to his French class without them.

Simon sat back in the chair and took a deep breath as Nick left. Things seemed to have moved very fast and he wasn't sure whether he had pushed it along too quickly. But then, the issue of bullying was important and shouldn't be brushed aside. He had a responsibility and had to exercise professional judgement. It was affecting Nick badly. He was pleased that his form teacher had suggested listening out for it and trying to catch it happening. Nick had looked somewhat relieved when she had said that.

He noticed the clock – not long before his next client. He wrote his notes in rough, deciding to write them out on his records later. He went over to the window and took a few deep breaths himself and then poured himself out some water.

Points for discussion

- How were the core conditions of empathy, unconditional positive regard and congruence present for Simon in this session?
- Nick is experiencing extremes in his reaction to the situation at school. What feelings are likely to be present for him that have not been voiced?
- How might your school experiences impact on your work with a young person who is being bullied?
- Was it appropriate to bring in the form teacher?
- How are you left feeling at the end of the session: towards Nick, towards Simon, towards the school?
- Write notes for the session.

CHAPTER 15

Counselling session 4: client adjusting to feeling different

Since the last session, things had moved on in the school concerning the bullying that Nick was alleging was occurring on a widespread basis. Simon did not know all of the details, but when he had arrived that morning Mrs Abbott had come to see him and informed him that the matter was now being addressed in the school, that it had been raised at assembly and that the teachers' awareness was now heightened on the matter. The school was adopting a policy of zero tolerance: anyone caught bullying would be disciplined and parents would be informed. It had all come about because she had herself spoken to her year head about it after having caught the kids who were giving Nick verbal abuse, in fact that very afternoon after his last counselling session. The year head had in turn mentioned it the following morning at a routine meeting that he had with the headmaster and at the next staff meeting it had been discussed.

Simon had been somewhat taken aback by the speed of things. His initial concern was for Nick, and what effect all this may have had on him. He had asked her about this and she said that his name was not involved. The two who had been caught giving him verbal abuse were being dealt with and it was being regarded as one incident among many that would be dealt with.

When she had left Simon was still wondering what effect it may have had on Nick, given his hesitancy in saying anything. But Nick wasn't due until lunch-time, so he had to wait to find out. He hoped that Nick would still come and feel able to trust the counselling relationship – well, he thought, that's a fancy way of saying will he trust me.

He next had a call from the teacher responsible for pastoral care, wanting a word at some point. At this meeting – hastily arranged between clients – Simon was asked if he would pass on any disclosures of bullying. Simon responded by pointing out the confidentiality and the right of the young person to decide on that, but that he would bring it up and discuss it. However, he emphasised that the child had a right to confidentiality and that there would be times when, in his professional judgement, maintaining focus on the client's therapeutic process of working with their experience would be more important than shifting focus to a discussion on whether the young person wanted to have the details passed on. The head of pastoral care accepted that, and they agreed to keep in touch on the issue in general terms.

Nick arrived on time. He looked pleased, which Simon found encouraging given his own anxiety about the effects of what had been happening in the school.

'You look pleased; is that how you are feeling? I've heard from Mrs Abbott already this morning and I understand things are happening.'

The counsellor, for reasons of transparency, makes clear that he is aware of what is happening and that he has had a conversation with the form teacher already. Making this visible to the client is a much healthier choice; it is more authentic and encourages openness.

'Mrs Abbott caught two of them having a go last Thursday, during the break. They were both hauled off and got a detention for it. They've both been less hassle since. And it seems like the whole school is talking about bullying.'

'The whole school? And you're getting less hassle?'

Nick nodded. 'Yeah. And it's like there seem to be more teachers around all of a sudden. They used to all disappear to the staff room, but now, well, they're just around more. It's really helping.' He was grinning.

'And you haven't had any hassle over it, but less hassle, yeah?'

'Yeah. And it feels good.'

'Mhmm, feels good not getting the verbal.'

Nick nodded again. 'And it got talked about at assembly yesterday, no, Tuesday. The headmaster really came on strong. Never seen him so, well, kind of angry I guess.'

'That felt good too?'

'Yeah, like someone's fighting back, you know, and that feels really good.' He was nodding from the chest up as he said it, clearly really pleased about it. 'Yeah, really good.'

'I'm pleased, but I was concerned when I heard how fast things had moved how it had left you feeling, given that you were hesitant on saying any of this to anyone else last week.'

Simon is acknowledging his reaction to what is happening, his pleasure that something is happening, but also the fact that it had left him concerned as to the effect on Nick. This communicates his warmth for Nick, that he thinks about his well-being beyond the session. It helps to encourage in Nick a sense that he is not invisible to people.

'Yeah, I know, but I'm glad now. It feels a relief . . . like, like . . .' Nick paused and thought about it. 'It's like not having to keep a secret; I don't feel I have to worry about it so much, I mean, you know, I feel kind of, I don't know, kind of ...' He struggled to find the right word, but couldn't seem to get it. He knew he was feeling different, not so worried, but didn't know how to describe it.

Emotional literacy can be a problem, and not just when working with young people. The counsellor can helpfully try to encourage the client to find words, or to describe feelings in other ways, or even suggest describing it in terms of what it is not like.

'Struggling to find the right word, yeah?'

Nick nodded his head. 'I just feel different.'

Simon had a word in his head, 'liberated', but wanted to help Nick find his own language. 'Different. I wonder, can you describe the difference?'

Nick thought about it. 'It's like, before I was always walking with my head down and, well, just always kind of edgy, you know. Now that's not there, at least, not all the time. Sometimes it is, but it's kind of not so intense. I feel, well, I feel less on edge.'

'Mhmm, less edgy, less on edge, less anxious, less head down.'

'And it's a good feeling. And I seem to be talking more to some of the other kids as well, and it's like something's happening.'

'Something helping you to talk to other kids?'

'Well, yes, but they also seem to talk to me, I mean, not everyone, but it feels different somehow. Feels like ...' Nick was still struggling to find the words, then the awareness struck him. Yes, that's it, that's what it is. 'I'm not feeling so alone.'

'Not so alone, like it's shared.'

'Yes but not just that. It's like something's happening and, yeah, I started it, didn't I?'

Simon nodded. 'Yes, you did.' He paused. It was good to see Nick grinning again. 'And how does that affect you?'

'Makes me feel kind of strong, somehow, like, yeah, I've kind of made a difference. Like I've made the teachers take notice of me, well, not me, but of something I wanted them to know. Yeah, that does feel good.' As he said that he sat up straighter in the chair and kind of shifted from side to side.

'Good feeling, huh, making a difference, realising you have some power.'

Nick was still grinning.

'Seems like a cause for celebration, Nick, you've fought back.'

'Yeah.'

Simon was aware of a concern as to whether this current climate in the school would last, but the fact that things had moved quickly seemed to be indicative that perhaps there was a strong, collective will present to address it. He was kind of curious as to what had been said at the assembly and decided he would check that out later if Nick didn't tell him. He didn't want to ask Nick; that was his agenda and he didn't want to make Nick feel he had to fit in with the counsellor's needs over his own.

It is an important feature of the person-centred approach to ensure that the client maintains as much autonomy as possible, and that they are enabled to experience the session as theirs, as the place in which they can be and talk about what is important to *them*.

Simon grinned back at Nick and waited to see what he would say next.

'And I told my parents.'

'You told your parents as well? How was that?'

'OK. I sort of thought I might after last week, but it was because Mrs Abbott caught Chris and Roger, it sort of, well, made me feel somehow more able to say something. But I still kept quiet until after Tuesday. I told them about the assembly.'

'Mhmm.' Simon noted how easily Nick was now saying the names of the two bullies.

'You want to know what I said?'

'I'm curious but it's up to you.' Simon smiled.

'Well, I said that the school was sorting out some bullying.'

Simon nodded.

'My mum wanted to know if I was OK. And that helped me to say that I'd been having problems, but that the teacher was addressing it. I told her what was being said – that was the really difficult bit. I got quite upset. And said that I was feeling better about it now.'

'So, that was quite an achievement, something that you hadn't been able to do before.'

Nick took a deep breath. 'Then she must have told my father when he came in 'cos he came up to my room and asked about it. I told him what had happened. "No one's hit you, though, or anything like that?" Typical of him. I told him no.'

Simon was struck by the 'typical of him', and said so.

'Yeah, well, Dad doesn't talk much about feelings. He started telling me about how to fight. He's done that before. I told him it wasn't like that and the school was dealing with it. He finally seemed to accept that and ruffled my hair before heading back downstairs.'

'Was that what you wanted?'

'Yeah, that's how he is. And he bought me a new game, came home with it last night. It's really great.'

'So, you told your mum, she told your dad, and you feel, what, OK about it now at home?'

Nick nodded. 'Yeah.' He paused. A thought struck him really forcibly. He'd had the thought before but somehow it really hit him. 'I hope it really has stopped.'

'That's a really difficult one, "Has it really stopped?"'

> Simon avoided saying that he thought it wouldn't happen again. That was simply a false reassurance and he had nothing to base it on other than hope and a wish to rescue Nick from this uncomfortable thought. No, he thought, what Nick is feeling is a very real concern and I need to be here for him as he encounters it.

'I really hope so. It had made me so miserable. Bastards. Still want them to get it. Still like to think of blasting them with a ray gun or something.'

Those bloody games, Simon thought again, putting ideas into kids' heads about how to deal with things, with people, with problems – blast them away. And his dad wants him to fight.

'That's the answer, is it, blast them away?'

'Yeah, I guess so. But maybe I won't need to, maybe the teachers'll do it for me. But I'd still like to.'

'Yeah, you'd still like to blast them away.'

'Blast them all away. You should have seen the headmaster. If he'd had a ray gun ...'

'Yeah?'

Nick held his hands up as though he was holding a ray gun and made noises indicating him firing it around the room at imaginary people.

'You'd have liked that?'

'Yeah, wasted 'em all. Let the rest of us get on in peace. Yeah. Bullies should be thrown out of school. They're a fucking pain in the arse.'

> Simon noted the sudden colouring of Nick's language and he guessed that some strong feelings were coming to the surface. He sought to stay with this process, using similar language himself and with some edge to his words, encouraging the climate in the room for further contact with, and expression of, those feelings.

'Mhmm, they're a fucking pain in the arse, and you've had enough of them, and you want them got rid of, permanently.'

'Yeah. They've been giving me grief since I've been at this school. I don't know why. I mean, why me, why me? Bastards.'

'Why you?'

'Dunno. Just started on me not long after I was here. Didn't say anything. Just tried to get away each time. That's what I did when it happened at my last school. Didn't stop them though.'

'So you tried to get away, same as you did at the previous school, but it didn't work.'

Nick shook his head. 'No. Should have fucking beaten the shit out of them, but I couldn't, didn't think, just wanted to get away. But that's what I should have done. Said something back, or something ...'

Simon was nodding; he realised that he had slipped out of counsellor role, but was thinking back to his own childhood memories, and how difficult it was for a child to fight back once they had been singled out.

'So that's how you see it now, that you should have said something, done something when it started, yeah?'

'Yeah, should have, but didn't. I don't want to be like that but I don't know how to be different. I'm really worried it'll happen again.'

'Nick, I can really appreciate how scary that thought is, but it doesn't have to be that way. We can learn from experiences, make changes, find other ways to be.'

Simon was aware of having stepped out of Nick's frame of reference. Yet it felt right to do so, somehow, to offer a perspective broader than that which Nick was experiencing. Yet he also knew that it might have been more therapeutically helpful to wait for Nick to make this recognition himself, even if it might take some time. After all, person-centred counselling was about providing a therapeutic space for someone to experience themselves more fully and openly. Nick was already finding a new way to be in response to the changes taking place in the school. Yes, he still carried doubts about himself, and probably would for some while. And those doubts were real and part of who he had become. But given more healthy relationships, and he believed person-centred counselling could be a crucial element to this, Nick and other clients could, and would, adapt and find ways to achieve more satisfaction in their lives and be less affected by 'conditions of worth' and the introjects that set them, us, everyone, up to be to some degree incongruent.

'You really think so?'

Simon responded very clearly, 'Yes, I do.' He thought about saying something more, and decided he would. He had no clear justification for this; it was a spur-of-the-moment idea in his head, and he decided to share it with Nick. 'You see, being verbally bullied caused you to adapt and think in a particular way about yourself, yeah?'

Nick nodded. He was looking at Simon, suddenly feeling really concentrated on what he was saying.

'Well, time now spent experiencing not being bullied, being listened to, being accepted, will help encourage you to adapt again with new ways to think about yourself.'

That made sense, Nick thought, yeah, he could see that. 'So I need to spend more time feeling listened to, yeah?'

Simon felt like he had told Nick what to do, and he could suddenly imagine him saying, 'My counsellor told me you have to listen to me more.' He felt an internal grimace at the thought.

'How does that feel to you, the idea of being listened to, taken seriously, feeling, like here, that you have done something that can make a difference?'

'It feels good. It make me feel, yeah, kind of big somehow, kind of, yeah, good. Yeah, makes me feel like I am someone.'

'Like you *are someone*.' Simon was aware of the emphasis he had placed on those two words.

'Yeah, and that's how I want to be, you know?'

'Mhmm, you want to be, to feel, you are someone.'

'And I don't want to walk around with my head down any more. So many kids here do, and they're the ones being bullied, you know. They're the sad and miserable ones, like me, well, like I was.'

Simon nodded. 'Yeah, that's not how you want to be any more.'

Nick shook his head slowly. 'No.' He went silent.

Simon sat and stayed with the silence. In a way it felt like the dialogue they had just had may have reached its own conclusion, but perhaps other thoughts and feelings had now arisen in Nick. The clock caught his eye; the session was coming to an end. He didn't mention it; he felt that Nick might be processing something and to mention the time might simply cut across him and stop him from saying something from within his own process. He waited. Nick stayed silent.

Another couple of minutes passed and Simon knew he had to mention the time. 'We don't have many minutes left, Nick, but I'm aware you seem deep in thought about something.'

Nick took a deep breath and let it out slowly. 'Just remembering how miserable I've been and I guess how close it still is. Feel like there's two "me"s – the sad and miserable one with his head down, and the . . . well, the me I am now.'

'Quite a contrast and still difficult to find the words to describe you as you feel now.'

'Feels good to be me now, though. And I've made a difference, haven't I? I've really shaken things up. I don't think I'll ever forget seeing old Doberman – sorry, that's what we call the headmaster, Mr Durman – never seen him so fired up. That felt good, that felt really good.'

Simon smiled. 'So, same time next week, Nick?'

'Yeah, definitely. See you then.'

With that Nick left, leaving Simon to ponder the session. Mr Doberman, he thought to himself, he liked it. Kids and nicknames for teachers. It led him back into some of his own memories, before bringing himself back into the present and turning to write up his brief notes on the session.

Counselling session 5: tired of it all, the client falls asleep

Nick rushed over to the counselling room. He had got delayed again over lunch but was just about on time. He didn't want to be late. Somehow it felt good being with Simon. He wasn't sure exactly why. It still seemed strange sometimes, to be sitting there, sometimes not knowing what to say, but always feeling that you were being listened to. He wasn't used to that. He didn't get listened to much at home. In fact, it had been a bit of a surprise that his parents had taken the bullying seriously, but they hadn't really said much about it since. That was how it often seemed. Sometimes he felt quite sad; they just seemed too busy doing what they wanted to do with little time for him. But then, well, he liked being on his own in his room, playing his games. He liked it . . . mostly. Sometimes he had to convince himself that he liked it.

The session began with Nick saying a little about how things were at school with the bullying. It seemed that the prefects had also been alerted and were also more active. It really did feel different and he was really pleased with what was happening. Simon again allowed him time to feel good about it. He'd tried to tell his parents how things had changed because of him, but he didn't really feel they had heard how important it was for him. 'That's nice, dear' wasn't really enough. Nick continued to elaborate on this theme.

'I just feel that sometimes they don't really know I'm there. I mean, I know they do, but in a way they don't, and that's hard. I just wish sometimes they'd give me a bit of time, be there for me a bit more.'

'Mhmm, yeah, if they could be there for you a little more it would feel so much more different, yeah?'

'It would.' Nick lapsed into silence and thought about an incident a couple of days ago. He'd got home and no one was home. That happened a lot. He kind of didn't mind, but it felt uncomfortable going into the house on his own.

Simon noticed that Nick looked lost in thought and allowed the silence to remain while he connected with whatever was present for him. After a minute or so he commented, 'You look lost in thought, Nick.' He spoke softly so as to try not to disturb Nick's train of thought too much.

'Hmm? Oh, yes.' He went back into silence.

Simon continued to wait, feeling somehow that there was some kind of unvoiced discomfort in the atmosphere. He couldn't quite put his finger on it, but it had arisen since Nick had entered in that silence. It persisted. He voiced it. 'Something feels uncomfortable to me.'

Simon expressed something present within his sphere of experience that he senses to be connected to what is present for Nick. He is not suggesting anything about Nick's experience, but owning what is present for himself. The person-centred counsellor may voice these experiences, they may not, depending on their professional judgement in the moment.

Nick took a deep breath and sighed. 'Yeah.' He paused. 'It's just that . . .' He didn't like criticising his parents, though he wasn't sure why; he heard so many of the other kids doing so about theirs. He hesitated.

Simon responded, 'It's just that . . .?'

Nick sighed again. 'It's like, I really wish my mum and dad were there for me more. I mean, I like time on my own, doing stuff, you know, but, well, I guess it would be nice sometimes to come home and someone be there and be kind of pleased to see me. But that doesn't really happen much.'

'Feels like no one's there for you?'

Nick nodded. He could sense some strange feelings inside himself, and he didn't like them. He felt . . . he couldn't really describe it, but he felt kind of strange, like his tummy was kind of moving, though it wasn't, and his arms suddenly felt heavy.

Simon somehow sensed that Nick was uncomfortable. He looked awkward all of a sudden. He guessed that what he had just said had touched something in Nick, but he didn't want to rush into making assumptions.

Nick felt weird and he didn't like it. He suddenly felt very tearful, and he wasn't at all sure why, but he was crying, and the tears were very hot in his eyes. His throat felt like it had a large lump of solid mud in it. It was all heavy and tight. He coughed to try and clear it.

Simon responded, 'Sounds like you could do with a sip of water', and he went to pour one from the tap.

Nick took it and drank. It was good to feel it, cool in his throat, but it didn't really make much difference. Still felt like he had this lump inside his throat which he couldn't get rid of. And his tummy was still feeling odd. He blinked and rubbed his eyes.

'Uncomfortable, huh?' was all Simon said in response.

'I sometimes wonder why they bothered having me, I really do. I mean, I . . . Oh, I don't know, what's the point.'

'You wonder why they bothered and what's the point anyway, yeah?'

Nick was silent again for a while. When he spoke he had clearly moved into another focus. 'I feel awkward with other kids.' He spoke quite quietly, as if it had been a really difficult thing to say. Simon only just caught the words. He reflected them back to convey that he had heard what Nick had said, using the same words, as it felt important for Nick to feel that he had been heard, but he didn't say them as a reflection. He said them with a sense of his own wanting to understand what Nick was experiencing.

'You feel awkward with other kids.'

It is important to differentiate empathy from reflection. Reflecting is a skill, and it is helpful, but it does not require any depth of experiencing or connection with the client. Empathy, however, requires a genuine sensitivity to the inner world of the client that the words are themselves reflective of, and an urge within the listener to want to understand. The counsellor is interested, genuinely striving to hear the client accurately and to check back with the client that what they have heard is as it was intended to be conveyed.

Nick nodded. 'I kind of don't know what to say.'

'Difficult finding the right words?'

Nick paused. 'Difficult finding any words. And that's just with the boys. With the girls it is even harder. It's awful. I feel so useless.'

In that moment Simon's heart went out to him. He remembered struggling with that as well. He always seemed to get his tongue tied up when he wanted to talk to a girl, though fortunately that had passed. He felt an urge to reassure Nick and realised that while that was partly linked to his own stuff, maybe it might be helpful for Nick as well.

'Awful, not being able to say what you might want to say.'

'I don't really know what I want to say, but I go over it, again and again in my head afterwards. I just keep replaying it, you know, and I get so frustrated with myself.' Nick felt wretched, useless. He doubted he'd ever get a girlfriend and that really worried him. But that felt too difficult to talk about. He'd feel too embarrassed.

'Yeah, it's frustrating to not know what to say, but then round and round it goes in your head, replaying it again and again.'

Nick looked at Simon. 'You know what I mean, don't you?'

Simon nodded. 'I don't know if I experienced the same as you, but I do know what you're talking about.'

'Does it stop, I mean, will I get over it?'

'That sounds really important. And yes, it does stop. But maybe you need to find ways to build up your confidence.'

Nick nodded. 'I do. I need to get involved in things. The music group's good, I've really got into that, and I do talk a bit there. We're learning different instruments and I'm sort of having a try at different instruments, see what I like. I kind of like the viola, don't know why, but it kind of feels good.'

Simon nodded. 'So something about the viola feels good, and being at that group is helping you talk a bit more.'

'It is, but it's difficult.' Nick was thinking back to the last lesson – well, it wasn't so much of a lesson as just what he had described, time for them all to mess around with instruments and get a feel for them. Some seemed to already know how to play things, and that made him feel awkward, but he kind of liked the viola. He liked the sound you could make, he could make. He'd never done anything like that and it had felt good. He thought, too, of how he'd mentioned it at home to his dad, but he'd just kind of ignored it, well, no, actually he'd said, 'What do you want to be doing that for. Won't get you on "Top of the Pops".' Nick had felt really upset but hadn't shown it. He'd gone to his room.

'Difficult. Bringing back memories?' Simon had noticed Nick drift off.

'Yeah, well, I like the sound it makes.' He went on to talk about his dad's reaction. 'Really upset me. Bastard.'

Simon sought to avoid a reaction. It was the first time Nick had expressed a really powerful feeling towards his father. He'd shown anger towards his mother in an earlier session, but no strong feelings for his father.

'Really got to you, yeah, really upset you. Bastard, huh?'

Nick had felt a surge of energy inside himself but now, hearing Simon speaking, that seemed to have gone as fast as it had arrived. 'Yeah, he's OK really. Just doesn't understand.'

> As soon as Nick acknowledges his anger towards his father, another part of himself cuts in and takes him to a different place in himself, a place where he is used to making excuses for his father not offering him what he wants or needs. He is moving through configurations, which outwardly might appear confusing and unpredictable, but in Nick's reality is him simply moving through the various parts of himself that have an angle on the topic of his relationship with his father. Others are likely to be present but are not emerging at this time.

'So part of you feels it's OK how he is, Nick, but another part gets upset and is angry.' Simon added the bit about angry. It wasn't a word Nick had used, but he had certainly conveyed it just then. He simply sought to make it visible as something he had felt Nick communicating to him.

'Yeah ... No. I mean, I don't know. I just wish he'd encourage me a bit, take an interest, anything. Just feels like they're not interested. Too busy.'

> Nick is flustered, perhaps by the introduction of the word angry, or maybe because of the language of 'parts' Simon has adopted, which was not how Nick described it. Simon is not being empathic; he is introducing a model to make sense of what is occurring, but it is only serving to confuse Nick. Better that he had simply acknowledged the different feelings that Nick has expressed.

'That sense of them being not interested and too busy, that's something you mentioned before, must be a big part of what you experience with them.'

Nick rubbed his nose. He had just got a furious itch. 'If only they'd talk to me, anything. But, well, apart from the bullying thing, and yeah, that was good, but it's not usually like that. I feel I'm like in a different world.'

'Like you're in a different world, to their world do you mean?' Simon sought clarification as he wasn't clear.

Nick nodded and sat back in the chair and closed his eyes. 'Parents.' He spoke the words with an air of deep resignation.

'Parents,' Simon responded, seeking to maintain a similar tone of voice. And acknowledged to himself that he was one of those as well.

Nick took a deep breath and somehow, while he still felt a bit depressed about it all, he also knew he had to do something about it. He hated feeling this way, but it was all too common. Ever since his mum had gone back to work a couple of years back, not that it had been that good before then. Childhood, he remembered, seemed to involve being sat in front of the TV with a video. Actually, he liked it at the time, but looking back, that was all he could remember. Didn't remember going out much. Occasionally went to the swings, but not very often. He didn't know why. His mum always seemed to have the curtains closed as well. He always closed his curtains in his room now. He didn't know why. It was just what he did.

'I get depressed sometimes, just feel, well, what's the point?'

'What's the point in . . . ?'

Nick shrugged his shoulders and tightened his lips. He was looking down and fiddling with his trousers again. Simon realised he hadn't been doing that since the bullying had begun to be addressed. 'Dunno.' Silence. 'Everything.'

'Everything?'

Nick shrugged again.

A thought shot through Simon's mind. Was Nick struggling to be with himself as a non-bullied person? Or was that too soon? Was the lack of preoccupation with the bullying leaving him more sensitive and aware of his reactions to his parents? He didn't know. It seemed too soon. Anyway, he put the thought aside.

'All seems pretty pointless, yeah?'

Nick was feeling very heavy in himself. He wasn't tearful any more; this was different. He felt heavy and stuck, like he was kind of in glue, sticky glue, and it was inside him. All yucky. Nick even found it hard to nod. He was aware of suddenly feeling incredibly tired. He yawned and was aware of how heavy his eyes felt. He yawned again, longer this time.

'Tired of it all, huh?'

Bodies can psychosomatically reflect aspects of thought and feeling. Outbreaks of yawning can indicate that the client is tired of what they have been talking about.

Yeah, Nick thought to himself, there were days when he was tired of it all. But he could get himself together gaming. He could forget it all when he was on his computer. It wasn't really a computer, but a computerised game player. He was yawning again.

'Persistent, huh?'

Nick nodded. He felt very tired. Felt like he just wanted to go to sleep.

'I'm so tired. I want to go to sleep.' He closed his eyes and drifted off.

Simon sat wondering what to do next. Yes, Nick was asleep. He heard a change in his breathing. He really wasn't sure what to do. He'd not had this happen before in a counselling session. Nick must be so tired. Was it just being tired of everything, or was he genuinely tired, from not sleeping well, or from staying up too late playing at his games? He sat there pondering and aware that time had passed. Nick was still asleep. In a real sense he wanted to let him sleep. It was obviously what he needed. But he didn't want to wake him up at the last minute, assuming he didn't wake up himself. Simon had looked at the clock and there were still 20 minutes or so of the session left. He decided to let Nick stay asleep for a bit longer.

> Simon has chosen to allow Nick to experience what clearly his organismic self is choosing. In a sense he is conveying empathy and respect for the client's clearly expressed need.

After almost ten minutes Simon decided he ought to rouse Nick, and give him some time to get his bearings and process what had happened. 'Nick,' he called softly, then a little more strongly, 'Nick, you've dozed off, time to wake up.' He decided not to touch him to wake him, aware that it might be unhelpful for Nick to awaken and find himself being touched. He wanted to bring him back with the minimum of invasiveness as possible.

'Hmm?' Nick roused himself slowly, opened his eyes and blinked, yawned and stretched. 'What happened?'

'You fell asleep.'

'Sorry.' Nick felt awkward.

'That's OK. You must have been really tired.'

Nick nodded. 'Guess I've not been getting to bed early.' He yawned again. 'What were we talking about?'

'Feeling tired about everything.'

Nick remembered. 'Oh yeah. I was, wasn't I?' He grinned, but a little sheepishly.

'Yeah, that's OK. Look, we've got a few more minutes before you have to go. Is there anything else you want to say today?'

Nick shook his head. He felt like he needed some fresh air. 'No. I think I'll head off. I need to get more sleep, don't I?'

'I think so. Seems like you're overdoing it a bit.'

The session drew to close. Nick left and Simon was still reflecting on the whole issue of what you do when a client falls asleep in the session, and a young person at that. He wondered if it had been a female client, would he have roused her sooner? He wasn't sure, but he thought he might have done. Just something he'd never thought of. He realised he needed to talk it through in supervision, which he would have before the next session.

Points for discussion

- What is your reaction to the school's reaction?
- The emotional literacy issue is an important one. It can be a challenge to work with a young person who does not have the language to describe their feelings beyond 'good', 'sad', 'pissed off', 'angry', etc. How would you handle this?
- Was it therapeutically helpful for Simon to start explaining the impact that the verbal bullying would have had on Nick and the effect that feeling listened to might now have?
- Describe the psychological process occurring within Nick bringing him to this sense of being 'two "me"'s'?

- How, in terms of his development, might Nick be affected by what he has described of his childhood so far?
- Discuss Simon's idea that a 'non-bullying sense of self' could be emerging within Nick.
- Was it appropriate for Simon to let Nick stay asleep? What might the implications of this be?
- Would it have been less appropriate had there been a different gender mix between counsellor and client?
- Write notes for these sessions.

CHAPTER 16

Supervision 2

'Well, it's all happening for Nick.'

'Tell me more.' Simon had Sarida's attention.

'He has told one of the teachers and the school has taken it seriously and is taking action, across the whole school, to come down hard on bullying. And it seems to be working.'

Sarida was curious. 'How did it happen?'

'Nick agreed to let his form teacher know, and she came into a session and he explained what was happening. It seems she passed it on and the next week the headteacher was talking about it in assembly, and there's been a real crackdown.'

'How did he come to agree to it?' Sarida was wondering how a teacher had ended up in the session.

Simon described what had happened.

'So you felt that Nick didn't feel pushed at all?'

'I don't think so. He seemed OK with it, although a little hesitant at the time. But he seemed to have realised that something had to change. It was affecting his schoolwork. But I think the fact that they listened and took him seriously has had a major impact.'

They went on to discuss this and in particular Simon drew attention to the fact that Nick had talked in the last session of not getting much attention from his parents, and how that left him feeling depressed and angry, particularly the incident with the viola and the music club.

'How does that affect you, Simon, I mean, hearing what Nick is experiencing?'

'Leaves me feeling bloody angry.'

'Bloody angry, really gets to you?'

Simon shook his head and took a deep breath. He knew he felt strongly about what had come to be called 'latch-key kids' – a horrible label. He wished there was a label that could be hung on the parents as well, for encouraging it. Well, in his view, it had been the government that had brought in the idea that mortgages could be based on two incomes, not one, so up went the house prices, and both parents end up having to work. And who suffers? The children. He described his thoughts and continued. 'And even when kids are at home, like Nick, they end up watching videos when they should be out playing. I suspect something is/was wrong with his mum. I don't know, but he remembers the curtains drawn all the time and not going out. Seems like something wasn't quite right, somehow. Anyway, I'm concerned what Nick is picking up from all of this. It leaves me feeling that counselling is going to be so important. And I think now he knows what it feels like to be listened to – with the school and the bullying – and with me, he's going to maybe begin to reassess some things. What the effect will be, I don't know. But his "what's the point" attitude worries me. I wonder if there might be, well there is, but I mean, whether there might be the possibility of serious depression given his struggle with social stuff.'

Sarida was aware that Simon had said a lot and she needed to clarify it for herself. 'So, something not right with his mum, leaving him sort of isolated? And he is, what sounds like, caught between feeling good about being heard and feeling bad about not being listened to.'

'Yeah, but he's maybe normalised the not being listened to, and it's affected his confidence and I'm sure his self-esteem as well. Why don't parents give their children time?' Simon sighed. 'Sorry. Just frustrates me.'

'Yes, and I think it's important that you acknowledge this to yourself, and what impact it may have on your relationship with Nick.'

Simon stopped and thought about it. 'Makes me feel for him more and maybe leaves me feeling more concerned as well.'

'Just more concerned, or unrealistically concerned?'

'Ouch!' Simon hesitated before continuing. He let out a deep breath slowly. 'Is it leaving me with unrealistic . . . ?' He thought further. 'I'm not sure.' Simon paused, collecting his thoughts and reflecting back over the sessions. 'I just have this nagging concern that he's isolated and is having to come to terms with some powerful factors that have shaped his sense of self. His early childhood is shady – literally. He was kept in the dark and I feel kept in the dark.'

'OK, so there's an area that's unknown, but could have had an impact.'

Simon nodded. 'Well, it has in a behavioural sense.' He went on to describe about Nick drawing his curtains.

'That trouble you?'

'Well, could be teenage stuff, but given the past I wonder. And he's struggling with relating to other kids and, yeah, again, could be teenage stuff, but . . .' Simon tightened his lips and shook his head. 'I don't know, I'm not feeling good about it. I can't really pin it down, but something doesn't feel good.'

'Maybe we can explore that now.'

The supervisor does not direct Simon into exploring it, but offers the opportunity, preserving a non-directive stance.

'OK.' Simon took a deep breath. 'Let me think about this, and get a sense of what is happening for me.' Simon tried to reconnect with that sense of unease, of it not feeling good. It was indistinct, but it was present. But he lost it and was back with an image of Nick. 'I'm back with the client, here. I mean, spending so much time on his own with those violent games, experiencing so much bully-ing, feeling inept – my word, not his – socially . . .' Simon paused. 'And yet he seems to relate easily to me. I mean, the dialogue seems to flow easily enough, and that kind of surprises me and yet it feels OK.'

A thought came to Sarida as she listened to Simon. 'I'm hearing different parts here, like there's the part of Nick that is relating easily to you in the sessions, and then there is another part that is the isolated and inept part, yet which has found a way of gaining satisfaction through the computer games.'

Simon nodded, and it reminded him of a thought he had had in that last session. 'And I'm wondering how his "bullied sense of self" and his maybe developing "non-bullied sense of self", if it isn't too soon for that, fit in as well.'

Simon was thinking of configurations within self, but he was aware that the parts he was describing were what he saw and experienced, and not necessarily those that the client might identify.

Configurations within self (Mearns and Thorne, 2000) are discrete sets of thoughts, feelings and behaviours that develop through the experience of life. They emerge in response to 'conditions of worth' and the symbol-isation of experiences, the Self being formed out of a constellation of config-urations with the individual moving between them and living them out in response to experience in the present.

'My guess is his non-bullied sense of self may predate all this but got suppressed when the bullying started, so maybe he will reconnect with it but it could be rooted in much earlier experience.'

'You mean like it may not have matured or developed in line with his develop-mental age?'

'Perhaps.'

'That could leave him quite vulnerable, but it does tie up with his not being able to face down the bullying, not that that's easy. But if he hasn't the developmental resources, enough of a strong sense of "I" as a robust individual, he's going to be flattened by it, isn't he?'

'Mhmm.'

'But in a way – oh shit – in a way that part of him has developed but it has taken a fantasy route, the computer games, where he feels powerful and strong and, as he says, able to waste all the bullies.'

'So you are saying he has developed but into some kind of fantasy world?'

Simon nodded. 'It's how much he knows it is fantasy, and how much of his non-bullied sense of self is finding expression through it and may be experiencing it so powerfully that it becomes, in effect, reality. And then if it is the only resource to satisfy that need for power, it become obsessive and potentially addictive. Nothing else will measure up to it.'

'I really hear your concern and I want to throw in the fact that we are fantasising here on an issue where fantasy is a major component, and we need to somehow not lose sight of that too. And I also feel some unease around Nick's development.'

'Yes, we are, well, I am fantasising here. I realise that. I don't know how Nick is processing stuff, but there is something very oppressive in terms of the influences upon him, and he needs ways of expressing himself. And the music seems important. He seems fascinated with the viola for some reason – says it is the sound he likes. I wonder if he could get expression into music. At least it's real, tangible, and so much healthier than violent computerised games all the time.'

'And we have to remember that he is making choices that are satisfying to him as he is at the moment. And we need, as person-centred counsellors, to allow him to feel that he is, as he is, warmly accepted as the young person that he is.'

Simon took a deep breath. 'Yeah. I'm losing sight of that. I'm getting caught up in my fantasy here. But I don't want to lose sight of it either.'

'You don't have to. It's a genuine concern. But it's yours. Not his.'

'No, his concerns are around feeling able to relate to other kids and getting his parents to give him some quality time.' Simon paused. 'He's stirring me up.'

'*He's* stirring you up?'

'OK, I'm stirring me up. Yeah. I need to acknowledge my feelings, thoughts and concerns, but keep them to myself. I know that. I guess I'm wondering about how Nick will be in the future and – yeah, I know what it is – I guess I'm feeling responsible, and a lot of responsibility, for trying to make a difference.'

'And you are. You've helped him find his voice over the bullying. You've helped him talk to his parents about it. You're helping him talk about stuff he's probably never talked about to anyone in his life. He needs a lot of warm acceptance, Simon, a really quality therapeutic relational experience to help him through the storms that are within him.'

Simon took a deep breath. 'You're right, of course. Thanks. Yeah, I am helping him, and I'm at risk of trying too hard.'

'I don't think it's about trying too hard; it's about whether you can stay with him as he is now, or whether your own fantasises will dominate the quality of your empathy.' Sarida was feeling quite strongly as she said that. It showed in her voice.

'And my fantasises may be real.'

'They might be, but you are there to listen to what is real for Nick and to be authentically present, and can you do that?'

Simon put his hand over his mouth. The 'and can you do that' really struck home. He nodded. 'Yes, I can, but only with my eyes open, and my heart open . . . and my mind open. And my ears. I have to listen to him, be there for him, and it could be rough. He's trying to find a voice, a sense of self with which to relate to the outside world. It's potentially as big as that, isn't it? Shit.' Another deep breath. 'I think I'm getting a better perspective on all of this now. This has been good. It feels like I'm getting clarity. I feel suddenly quieter, like a storm has passed in me, a kind of raging at things, but that's passed. I feel clearer.

I feel ready to be that companion for Nick, if he'll take me on that journey with him.' Simon was nodding his head. He could feel tears in his eyes. 'I want to be on that journey, Sarida, I want to help him through all this and find his way forward. And I know that I don't know what the outcome will be, but if I can give him warm acceptance, keep empathic to his world and be authentically present, and keep psychological contact with him, then I know it will have a therapeutic impact.' Simon stopped again.

Sarida was nodding. 'And I know you can do that, Simon, but sometimes our anger and our caring and concern causes us to lose that simple human-to-human connection.'

'My head went overtime on me and left my heart behind, Sarida, at least that's how I make sense of it now. I remember reading a little phrase a long time ago, and it's always stuck with me, "The head directs, the heart connects." '

'Connections . . .'

'Connections and relationship, that's what it is all about, isn't it, healthy connections and right relationship? Love, the greatest healing force in creation.'

'And yet a word we seem to shy away from using. And who do we begin with in loving?'

Simon smiled. 'Where we always have to begin any journey, with ourselves.'

Counselling session 6: a new friend but home life makes Nick sad

Simon had been feeling a lot more at ease with himself after that last supervision session. It never ceased to amaze him just how affected he could be from his clients and how helpful it was to talk it through, often discovering deeply held thoughts and feelings that had been previously hidden from view. 'Keep it simple, keep it heartfelt' was the phrase that had come into his thinking as he had left that session, and it was still very much present for him now as he awaited Nick's arrival.

Nick knocked on the door and Simon called him in as he moved towards the door himself. Nick appeared. He grinned. 'Hi.'

'Hi there. You look pleased with yourself.'

'Yeah, I am. It's been a good week. No bullying, and I seem to be beginning to get some friends. Starting to talk to people a little more, and it feels good though still a little weird.'

'So, big changes, Nick.'

'Yeah. Felt I needed to at least try a little harder and, well, it kind of happened out of that music club. I was messing about with some instruments and so was this other lad, Ben, and well, somehow it felt kind of easy. Anyway, yeah, felt good and we've kind of got to doing some stuff after school yesterday, and yeah, I feel a little easier. He lives near me so, yeah. It's good.'

'So, kind of just happened when you were messing about.'

'Yeah. So, yeah . . .'

'Mhmm.'

Nick had lapsed into silence. It did feel good being with Ben. He seemed to be quite a character really, into all kinds of stuff. Just felt good being around him. Nick started to talk a bit more about what he was doing at school. He somehow wasn't sure what to say but he kind of felt he wanted Simon to know more about him. It felt good talking about the subjects he was doing. He was concentrating better now. He didn't play the computer games quite so late, well, not every night. But he was sleeping easier, didn't have so much on his mind, though he still felt edgy at times.

Simon listened to what Nick had to say, acknowledging to himself that the bullying had probably left him maybe more sensitive in some ways, and he hoped that would pass given time. He stayed with what Nick was telling him, checking out as he spoke that he was understanding him right. It didn't feel too much like therapy, more like a conversation, but he felt OK with that. He realised that Nick probably hadn't talked quite like this to many people, maybe not to anyone, so his listening to what he had to say was in truth a therapeutic intervention.

Nick moved on to talk a bit about the bullying at the primary school. It seemed to have developed because when he had joined the school, his parents having moved into the area, he didn't know anyone, and because his mother didn't really mix with anyone he never got to know the other kids too well. He had found it hard to settle and make friends, and found himself being picked on. He had had a miserable time and had been glad to leave when his parents moved a few years later. But it had happened again. Now, though, he was glad it seemed to be over. And he still felt good about having been the one who had really made things happen.

He told Simon how some of the classes had taken on the bullying theme. In art they had painted anti-bullying posters. In English they had been asked to write a story on the theme. It had all helped make a difference. Some of the posters had been exhibited along with some of the stories.

Simon could feel the enthusiasm in Nick's voice. He wondered if he was witnessing a social activist in the making, someone who had discovered that their voice could make a difference. You never can tell, he thought to himself, how these kind of experiences can get internalised. He clearly recognised that it had given Nick quite a buzz, and set against his family experience of getting little attention it must stand out even more.

As Nick spoke, Simon was aware of feeling relaxed. That last supervision session had made a difference. It felt good listening to what Nick had to say. He thought about how much his parents were missing by not really communicating with him. Nick was bright and he could speak clearly and freely – something that perhaps he had not had much experience of, never feeling confident enough, but these few sessions of therapy seemed to be having a huge impact.

It was well into the second half of the session when Nick suddenly said, 'But I still feel sad as well.'

'Sad as well?' Simon waited for Nick to elaborate.

'You know, not being able to talk to Mum and Dad. They don't really understand me, you know, and I wish I could make them listen to me.'

Simon nodded. 'Yeah, if they'd only listen . . . and I'm wondering what it is you'd want to tell them, Nick.'

Nick thought for a moment. 'Just ordinary stuff, what I do at school, what I'm learning, how I feel I've changed and how I want to make more friends and stuff, you know?'

Simon nodded. 'Maybe you will start to tell them more, and maybe they will begin to listen.' As he said it he wondered if that was a really helpful response. It felt more like he was rescuing Nick from feeling what he was feeling.

Nick was shaking his head. 'I don't think so. I really don't think they'll ever really understand me, you know? They just care about what they're doing and they kind of fit me in – that's how it seems.' Nick went on to talk more about life at home, how his father seemed to go out most evenings down the pub, and his mum watched TV, and usually drank her way through a bottle of wine. They didn't seem to spend much time together. At weekends, dad went to football. His mum did stuff round the house. He didn't like football. Didn't see much point to it.

'Ben's not into football either. Likes to just mess around, and hang out, you know. Says he goes up to town at weekends and I'm going as well this weekend. Mum won't mind. She never takes much notice where I am and what I'm doing when I'm home so I don't suppose she'll be bothered if I go out.'

'She won't be bothered then, and you want to get out?'

'Yeah.' He nodded his head, 'Yeah, it'll be good.'

Time was nearly up and the session began to draw to a close. The next week was half-term and so there wouldn't be an appointment for a couple of weeks. Simon agreed to see Nick the following week. As Nick left, Simon noticed that he still felt at ease. It had been a good session. Nothing hugely deep and upsetting, although Nick had mentioned his sadness. Generally it had seemed quite a chatty session. He had enjoyed hearing more about Nick's interests at school. Somehow it brought more of him to life. He felt he was relating to more of him and that felt more satisfying.

So, he thought to himself, half-term approaches and Nick has made a friend and is planning to get out and about. He seems to be really taken with Ben, he thought. Ah well, good for him to get some social experience. Could be the making of him. He could feel in himself that he was looking forward to seeing Nick again at the next appointment and hearing all about it.

Counselling session 7: the client does not attend

Nick couldn't face going to see Simon. He had had a horrible time. Things had gone really wrong with Ben, and he had learned some really hard lessons. They were still sort of friends, but he wasn't so comfortable with him any more. He had decided earlier that day that he wouldn't go to counselling. He sort of wanted to, wanted to talk about everything, but he felt ashamed. He didn't feel he could tell Simon and he didn't think he could sit there and not tell him. So he had decided not to go. Instead he had taken longer over lunch and gone out with some other kids that he had got to know a bit more from the music club. Ben wasn't one of them.

Simon had sat waiting for Nick until about 15 minutes into the session. By then he had begun to suspect that he wasn't going to make it. Nick had been late before, but not this late. He didn't know why. Usually if a child was ill he was told, so he guessed it wasn't that. He didn't want to ask questions; Nick had a right to privacy and, well, it wasn't easy to maintain confidentiality, but he tried to ensure that only those who needed to know – the teachers whose classes a client was missing – were aware that they were attending counselling.

He waited a while longer, dipping into a counselling journal and reading about how many more counsellors there now were in schools. Good thing, he thought, so many youngsters have so much to cope with, so much pressure on them. He thought back to his own childhood. He smiled. Yes, he thought, I'm old enough to be able to say I had a childhood. Out to play, hardly ever at home. No one really that worried about safety, at least not in the countryside where he had been brought up. Different world, he thought. He couldn't remember advertising aimed at him to have this, buy that. Life seemed simple really. You made your own fun. You'd all meet up, play games. He remembered, what was it called – different areas had different names for it. He couldn't remember, but he knew it involved everyone hiding and someone having to find them and when they'd found a person they had to get back to a central point and call their name. Meanwhile, anyone else who was hiding, if they could get to the pole or whatever before their name was called, could release everyone who was 'captured'. Simple game, kids everywhere hiding all around and about, and then there'd be a frantic rush, trying to get to the centre.

Now, he never seemed to see kids playing. Endless shopping for the latest fashion. How the marketing executives had really got a grip on youth culture. Or time spent indoors, electronic entertainment, all hype. Or else it was boredom. He shook his head. OK, not every young person was at either end of this polarity, but many were – all or nothing, a classic mindset for addiction. He could see how kids could get conditioned into non-stop stimulation as the normal. Some would maybe then get into drugs to slow themselves down with suppressants –heroin, cannabis, alcohol; others would try to keep themselves running high – amphetamine, ecstasy, cocaine. He glanced at the clock. Oh well, he thought, Nick isn't going to make it now. He wrote him a note offering another appointment the following week and hoping he was OK. He took it down to administration who would put it in the register for the next morning.

Points for discussion

- How might his own parenting skills impact on Simon's attitude towards Nick's parents? How might this have been addressed in supervision?

- What are your feelings for Nick at this time? How would you describe him to someone who had never met him? What are the key aspects of his nature and experience of life?
- Evaluate the accuracy of Simon's empathy in the session Nick attended.
- What are your reactions to Simon's thoughts as he waited for Nick when Nick did not attend?
- Are your feelings towards Nick's non-attendance different now to what they were when he did not attend the first session? What is your speculation as to the possible reasons for his not attending?
- Write notes for the counselling sessions.

CHAPTER 17

Counselling session 8: problems and Nick is grounded

Simon was smiling as he heard Nick knock the door. He was ten minutes late. The door was open, but he called Nick in.

'Hi. How're things then?' As soon as he had said the words Simon was struck by Nick's expression. It was a total contrast to the last time he had seen him.

Nick sat down and said nothing. He was looking down. He mumbled that he was sorry he was late.

'That's OK. Looks like things aren't too good, Nick.'

Nick continued to stare down. He now wished he hadn't come. He felt bad about himself, ashamed, miserable. Didn't know what to say. Could feel himself retreating into himself. Didn't want to speak, just sat, continuing to stare down.

Simon sat with a huge sense of discomfort. Everything seemed suddenly so awkward and difficult. He didn't know why and he pushed aside the temptation to start speculating to himself. Nick was here and clearly not happy about something. So he respected his silence and stayed holding his feelings of warmth for Nick, and his acceptance that if he was to talk about what had happened it would be when he was ready to do so.

Time passed. The silence remained.

> Silences can be a feature of working with young people. Sometimes the young person does not have the words to describe a feeling; sometimes they don't know how to talk about personal experiences with an adult. The person-centred counsellor will want to respect the client's right for silence, but will also want to be ready to support and enable the client to speak if they want to but are experiencing a block from doing so.

Simon was aware of feeling uncomfortable. Was it his discomfort? Yes, of course it was; he was experiencing it. It might be in response to what he perceived Nick to be experiencing, but it was present within him as he sat and watched him. He didn't voice it. It didn't seem appropriate to self-disclose and take Nick's attention away from his own experience and into what was present for the counsellor.

Nick could feel his heart pounding and was sort of sweating. He didn't feel good. What was Simon going to say? He really liked him, but he'd messed up and everyone had been having a go at him. He couldn't face that happening again. Simon was important to him. He couldn't bear the thought that he might get angry with him, start telling him off. He hated people having a go at him. Made him feel like he did when he was being verbally bullied. He didn't want to face that. It was why he hadn't come the previous week. Oh shit, he thought, I wish I hadn't come. I want to speak and I don't want to. He took a deep breath and sighed. He closed his eyes and felt a wave of nausea pass through him. He really did feel sick. He hadn't eaten much for lunch, kind of pushed it round the plate. His stomach had been churning. He took another deep breath and sighed again. He heard Simon speak.

'Lot going on for you, Nick.'

That's an understatement, he thought, but he still said nothing. He could feel his heart really thudding now in his chest and his throat had gone really dry. His arms felt heavy; his head felt sort of strange. He felt really shaky. He knew he was going to be sick, and he got up and headed for the sink in the corner of the room. He only just made it in time. He wretched up what must have been the breakfast he had forced himself to eat that morning – thankfully he hadn't eaten very much. His mouth tasted awful and he ran the tap to clear it away. Simon had come over and was rubbing the top of his back.

'You OK, Nick?'

'I think so. I need some water to wash my mouth.'

Simon took a glass from the drainer and filled it with cold water.

'Better to sip it, maybe just wash your mouth and spit it out. Drink too much and it might set you off again.'

Nick was already sipping the water and spat it out; the tap was still running. He repeated the process three or four times until he felt he could live with the taste in his mouth. He then tentatively sipped and swallowed. It stayed down. 'I think I'm OK now, but I do feel hot.'

Simon nodded. 'Yeah, it can leave you hot, and sometimes cold. Do you want to go back to the chair, or stay here for a bit, or get some air at the window?'

'I'll get some air.' Nick went over to the window. He still felt really wobbly and a bit spaced out. He had started to go cold now. He moved away from the window and back to the chair.

'You OK to continue, or what do you need to do, Nick?'

'I just need to sit for a moment, get myself together a bit.'

'Something didn't agree with you, needed to get it out.'

Hmm, thought Nick in response, that's not all I need to get out, but shit it feels difficult to say. He sat in silence again. Simon stayed with the silence. He had tightened his lips and without realising it had also tightened his jaw. He realised that it was aching. He relaxed it a little.

'Some difficult things to get out, to talk about, huh? I don't know what has happened Nick, but I really do want to listen to you and maybe help make sense of it.' Simon spoke as he felt.

What Simon has said can seem a bit 'counsellor-speak', and when it is spoken as a technique rather than as a genuine expression of what is present for the counsellor, that is how it is likely to be received. Counsellors have developed a certain language: 'Seems like . . .', 'I am wondering . . .', 'So what you are saying is . . .', 'Can you tell me more about . . .'. They can be helpful, but they can also end up sounding like a record with the needle stuck in the groove (for those of us who remember records with grooves!). The person-centred counsellor wants to use words that reflect, genuinely and sincerely, what they are experiencing. They will only want to say 'I wonder if . . .' when they truly are wondering, and 'Seems like . . .' when something really does seem to them to be a certain way. 'I hear what you say' is another counsellorism that doesn't convey anything to the client that demonstrates that they really have been heard.

He sounded really genuine to Nick, as he sat in silence. But how would he react? He'd done something so bloody stupid. It had been awful. He'd felt so scared. Sitting there, waiting for his parents. His father, so angry. Hadn't tried to understand. And now he was grounded, no computer games for a month. He'd had an awful week. Awful. But he stayed silent. He didn't know where to begin, how to begin, and he didn't want to risk Simon getting angry. After all, every other adult had; why should he be any different? He kept his silence.

Simon remained silent as well. He was aware of feeling stiff in his back. He realised he had been sitting quite tensed up. He moved his shoulders to free himself up a little. He could feel a few cracks in his back as he did so. He realised his own shoulders had been up with the tension. He sought to relax them, drop them down and just feel a little looser. He shifted his posture, leaning forward slightly, resting his forearms on his knees.

'Gonna risk telling me? It'll feel easier once you've said it.'

Nick opened his mouth but no words came out. He closed it again. He stayed looking down. He felt so ashamed. In many ways he couldn't believe what had happened, seemed like some dream, some horrible dream that had become a nightmare. He didn't want anything to do with Ben, ever again. He'd got him into trouble. He blew air into his cheeks; he still had his head down. He closed his eyes. He realised he wanted to say something to Simon, he wanted someone to understand, to listen, but he was an adult and he just wasn't sure. He felt he deserved to be told off. He was useless, waste of space. Yeah, 'Nicko the thicko' – they were right. Couldn't get anything right. He realised he was shaking his head.

Simon had also noticed the head movement. 'Hard to believe, huh?'

Was there such a thing as 'speculative empathy'? Simon put the thought aside and waited again. At least he felt he was reminding Nick that he was there, but it didn't seem that anything he was saying was in any way enabling Nick to find his voice. Maybe it was going to be a largely silent session, Simon thought. Well, so be it, but he was concerned at what the effect would be therapeutically if Nick went away feeling unable to say what he might be desperate to say. Yet to help him too much might leave him feeling undermined, that he needed someone else to help him. Yet, plainly, he did need help. Something was happening for him, something had happened, and he wasn't saying. But he was still here, sitting. He could have left. He hasn't; something is keeping him here, Simon thought to himself. So he maintained his feelings of warmth and unconditional acceptance of Nick. He was a great believer that attitudes of heart and mind, even when they are not voiced, can still affect the atmosphere and the relationship.

Nick was thinking back over the counselling sessions. Simon had listened to him. He had felt as though he cared. But he didn't want to make Simon feel bad about him. He didn't want that. He liked to come here because Simon seemed to feel good about him, took him seriously. Would he ever do that again? He'd fucked up, he thought. Someone who listened and took me seriously, now look what I've done. Fucked up. He took another deep breath and sighed again.

Simon reflected it back, himself taking a deep breath and sighing as well. 'Not easy, is it?'

Nick shook his head.

Simon sensed that they were at least communicating now, however minimal it was. The idea of asking him again if he felt OK after having been sick went through his mind, but that was a distraction. He let that go.

'No.' Simon sat and waited again.

Nick took a deep breath; his heart was pounding again and he could feel himself feeling weird again. He had to say it. He couldn't keep holding it in. Maybe it would be better once he'd said it. But that didn't take away the feeling that he'd let Simon down. But he had to say it. He swallowed and reached over to the glass of water. His hand was a bit shaky. He sipped some and swallowed again. He held the glass in his lap, still looking down.

'Got caught stealing some stuff.'

Simon felt for Nick in that moment. He closed his eyes momentarily and tried to imagine what anguish he must have been going through, struggling to say it, and having to face people having been caught.

'Must have been awful, getting caught.'

Nick nodded. That wasn't the response he'd expected at all. 'Won't do it again.'

'I'm sure you won't.'

He hadn't expected that either. Now he was feeling confused. He'd expected Simon to say something like, 'Oh Nick, what have you done?', or 'What the heck did you do that for?', or something to make him feel even worse. That's what everyone else had done to him. But he hadn't.

Simon was seeking to stay with and empathise with Nick's feelings as he was communicating them. It must have felt awful and he felt sure that given the reaction to it, as reflected in his struggle during the session, it was highly likely he wouldn't do it again.

Simon thought about asking Nick if he could tell him what happened, but he held back a little longer, waiting to see if Nick would be able to initiate this for himself.

'I thought you'd have a go at me.'

'Mhmm, what, thought I'd be angry?'

Nick nodded, very slowly.

'No.' Simon was genuine. How could he feel angry? The kid had done something really stupid and boy did he know it. Getting angry wasn't going to help. Nick needed understanding. He probably hadn't got much of that over the last few days. He continued, 'I'm not feeling angry.' He paused, then continued, 'I'm feeling sad that you've had such a tough time. Must feel awful.'

Nick nodded again. This time not so slow. He sighed and looked up, but only briefly. 'It was so stupid and it was that bastard Ben's fault.'

'Ben, that you mentioned last time? All his fault?'

'Yeah.' Nick could feel the urge to continue now. His heart didn't seem to be thumping quite so much. 'We went up to town and I didn't know. He told me he'd done it loads of times. Went into this sweet shop and we nicked some sweets. Got away with it. Felt so good, walking along the street eating them. Yeah, that felt so good.' Nick was kind of reliving it but not really. The same feelings weren't there. It all seemed unreal somehow now. He knew it had happened, but, well, just didn't give him the same feelings when he thought about it.

'Mhmm. Felt good, yeah.'

'Did then, not now.'

Simon nodded. 'The good feeling gone now.'

Nick took another deep breath and again tightened his lips, like he was trying to stop the words coming out. But they did nonetheless.

'He said, "Let's go in here", I don't know, some big store. Told me he'd nicked toys from there in the past. I didn't feel comfortable with the idea, but, well, he was my friend and I really didn't want to say no. Didn't want to appear useless or afraid or anything like that. So we went in. He told me to just put things in my pocket, small things. I saw these two little cars. Not really interested in them, but felt I had to take something, to kind of prove myself. Just put the second one in my pocket and the man put his hand on my shoulder. He was a security guard. He'd noticed me. Guess I'd looked guilty. I tried to run but he held me back. Ben was nowhere to be seen. He'd buggered off. Bastard. And I didn't want those cars. I tried to say it was a mistake but I got taken off to this room and someone else came and they told me off, and then they asked for my parents' phone number. Mum was working that afternoon – Dad was at the football. They asked where she worked. They called her. She came over about 15 minutes later. She was angry.'

Nick stopped speaking. He could still see her vividly in his memory. 'She was fuming. Had a real go. Apologised to the man who was there with me and the woman who had come in with him. I felt awful, felt so, so hurt and ashamed and . . . I just wanted to run away and hide.'

Simon acknowledged the feelings of awfulness, and hurt and shame. Nick continued.

'I got taken back home and sent to my room. I just sat there feeling awful still, knowing she'd tell Dad and that he'd go ape-shit.' Nick closed his eyes. 'He came back and was furious. Told me I was a fucking little thief and that I'd brought shame on Mum and himself. He kept going on about what people must think of *them*, how *they* couldn't go in that shop again because of me. He just kept on and on and on. And, yeah, I did fuck up and . . .' he shook his head, 'feel like shit.'

'Yeah, feel like shit after your dad had a go at you as well.'

'I've never stolen anything in my life, not before, never. But he wouldn't believe me. Told me I was a liar as well as a thief. Just kept going on and on.'

'No let up, huh, called you a liar and thief and just wouldn't believe anything you said.'

'I tried to say it hadn't been my idea. He said he didn't care whose idea it was; I was the one that had done it. And it set him off again.' There were tears in Nick's eyes. 'I hated it. Hate him. Hate myself. Hate them all.' He dissolved into tears.

Simon's heart went out to Nick. Yeah, he had done something stupid, he knew he was wrong, and yes, he needed to be told off, punished in some way, but all this on top of Nick's sensitivity and low self-esteem linked to the verbal bullying. Of course he was going to react badly to it.

'Yeah, hate everyone.' Simon didn't add any more. He waited and just felt what he felt for Nick, who was still crying.

'I don't know what to do, I feel horrible.' The tears began to subside and Simon passed him a tissue. Nick took it, wiped his eyes and blew his nose.

Simon had a sense of how alone Nick was with it all, but he also felt glad that he had been able to voice it in the session. He'd struggled with it not just during the session, but hadn't come last week. Must have been battling with these feelings ever since it had happened. And while he didn't want to slide into sympathy, he nevertheless recognised that here was a young person, sensitive and hurting about something which was not being acknowledged.

'Can't have been easy carrying these feelings around . . .'

Nick was shaking his head.

'. . . but I'm glad you've told me. Maybe it'll help to take a bit of the pressure off.'

Nick nodded and took a deep breath. 'You're not reacting like I expected. Everyone else was cross. You don't seem cross with me. I don't know why.'

'Sounds like my reaction has confused you?'

Nick was nodding, and sniffing. He had taken another tissue.

'Hey, I care about you, Nick, and I don't like seeing you hurting like this.' Simon was speaking from the heart. It felt incredibly important somehow in this moment to be genuine and to not hold back. He knew the risk might be further confusion for Nick, but he wanted to communicate that he cared about him. 'You've achieved so much recently and, yeah, I want to help you build on it and when you are ready move on from what's happened.'

Nick was still bemused. People didn't listen to him, didn't take him seriously. He was back in the self-doubt that had been so much a part of his life before he had started coming to counselling. And yet, here he was, and Simon was listening. It seemed that somehow it was OK here to talk about these things, to admit to having fucked up. He still felt miserable and yet somehow he didn't now feel quite so upset as he had a few minutes ago. 'I wish things were different at home.'

'Things you'd like to change at home?' As he said it Simon realised he hadn't really empathised; he had shifted the focus from Nick's experience of *wishing* to the *things* he wanted to change. But he had voiced his response now.

'Lots. I just wish they'd be on my side some of the time. They're just not interested. I hate going home and I hate being at school. And now I'm banned from my games and I've got nothing.' It all felt so bleak.

Simon had this overwhelming sense of emptiness, and a sense of his own anxiety as to what Nick would do. He still had a few weeks without his games and he knew how important they had been.

'Wish I was dead.'

Simon was alert. OK, he thought, don't panic, may be a passing thought. There may not be any suicidal planning, just a turn of phrase to express what he is feeling.

'Wish you were dead, or wish everything was different?'

'It's not going to be different. My parents won't change.'

'So nothing will change, nothing will be different?' As Simon said this, he could feel the urge to say, 'But the school's changing.' He didn't voice it. He stayed with what Nick was communicating.

Nick took another deep breath and sighed. 'What's the point. I even get myself a friend and he fucks me up, bastard.' Nick really did hate Ben. He really wanted to kick the shit out of him, but he hadn't seen much of him that week. But he was going to get him.

'You really hate Ben, don't you?' Simon was aware that they had moved away from the 'wish I was dead', but he felt he needed to stay with Nick. To go back might simply convey his own anxiety more than anything else, but he would check it before the end of the session.

'Fucking do. It's all because of him. And I didn't want those cars anyway, not really. Just wanted to do what he did, you know. No more of that.'

'So you'll not be doing that again. Hard lesson, huh?'

Nick nodded. 'Yeah, never do that again.'

Simon stayed silent and waited to see what Nick would want to say next. He was aware of feeling a lot of respect for Nick, for his being honest about it all in the session. He felt he wanted to honour that. 'Nick, it must have been so difficult coming here and telling me what you have told me. I just want to say I appreciate your honesty in all of this, you know? I genuinely mean that.'

Nick glanced up. 'Thanks. It wasn't as bad as I thought it would be, though it's been bloody awful too.'

'Yeah. Look, I'm aware that the time is nearly up, and I do want to check that you're OK to head off. I mean, you talked about wishing you were dead and wanting everything different. Were you serious about wanting to end it all?'

Nick shook his head. 'No, just get like that sometimes. Get to wondering what it would be like if I was dead, you know? I just wonder about it sometimes, what'll happen. Don't go with all the God stuff and heaven, but sometimes, recently, I've just been wondering. Maybe having time, not having my games, just thinking.'

'But no intention to actually find out?'

Nick shook his head. 'No, life may be shit but, no, nothing like that. I'll serve my month's sentence and then I'll really be up for it. Feel like I want to blast everything in all the games, you know, really let 'em have it. That'll feel good. Just got to wait I guess.'

Simon nodded, yeah. 'But if you did feel that way, would you promise to tell someone, your mum or a teacher, or me?'

Nick nodded. 'Think I'd tell you and maybe Mrs Abbott. Don't think Mum'd take me seriously, not the way things are at the moment anyway.'

'Yeah, I realise things are different at the moment, but she did take you seriously about the bullying. But you're the one at home and who knows what it feels like at the moment. But she did listen before.'

Nick nodded; he'd forgotten about that. 'Maybe, but that's not where I'm at. I want to put this behind me and, yeah, you're right, at least things have changed around here a bit.'

'How's your tummy now?'

'OK. Don't know what that was, maybe something I ate?'

'Maybe, but maybe all the anxiety about coming here got to you as well. But look after yourself, yeah, try and keep drinking water and, yeah, try and take it easy this afternoon. You feel OK for lessons?'

Nick nodded. 'Yeah. Thanks.'

Nick got up and headed out the door. 'Thanks.' He seemed quite thoughtful to Simon as he left. Simon was aware of how he had been left feeling – quite drained. What a session. So much struggle to tell him about what he had done, the shame, the anger with his friend, and his parents, and with himself. Being sick, so much upset, death and off he's gone to his lessons saying he's OK. And people say that counselling's just a case of spending your time listening to people. He took a deep breath himself and went out for a walk. He felt he needed that before he jotted down his notes, to clear his head and just get his own focus back.

Supervision 3

'Nick's having a tough time at the moment, Sarida, I was quite concerned at the last session. A real contrast to the previous session when all seemed to be going well.'

Sarida asked him what had been happening and Simon explained about the new friend, Ben, and how it had gone wrong with the theft of the toy cars, how it had affected Nick and his ongoing difficulty communicating with his parents. Also how everyone's reactions seemed to have fed into his low self-esteem, leaving him wondering what the point of it all was. He highlighted, as well, the theme of death that had emerged towards the end of the last session.

'Not unusual, that, there comes a time often around his age when young people become aware of the reality of death. It can be quite disturbing and upsetting for some. But you mentioned as well that he had wondered if he was better off dead?'

'Yes, and I did reflect that back but he moved on. I highlighted it again at the end of the session, and he confirmed that it was just a way he got into sometimes. He indicated he wasn't serious about ending it all and then he was into talking about death. Said he would serve his month's sentence – banned from playing computerised games which seem such an important part of his life – and then move on. Said he was looking forward to it, was going to "blast everything" I think he said. He really uses them to release the build-up of feelings and frustrations that he has. In a way it's good that he has something, but I'm still concerned about it as the only way he has. He doesn't seem too interested in sport so I don't think he's burning energy that way. I don't know, I know it's me, I just get frustrated with kids getting so into these things – it all seems to be about killing, you know. I just can't see it's healthy, plus staring at the screen for so long, and the risk of repetitive strain injuries. But maybe I'm just getting old and cranky!'

'That how you feel, old and cranky?' Sarida couldn't help but smile.

'Sometimes. But it does worry me, and sometimes I feel I'm the only one on the planet who's concerned.'

Sarida nodded. 'I appreciate your concern, and I want to check out what impact it might be having on your relationship with Nick. I mean, perhaps the most important thing in his life is something that you have real concerns about. Could be that your feelings have quite an impact on, perhaps, the quality of your empathy?'

Simon thought about it for a moment. 'He hasn't really talked about the games in any great depth, but he does refer to them. I'm just wondering about how I react.' Simon asked himself the question, 'Do I lose him in my own reactions?' He thought about it, but he didn't think so. 'I think I can stay with him on this, but then, if he really got into detail, then I'm not so sure. I think I'd feel I'd need to own what I would be feeling.'

'Which would be.'

'That maybe there's a world beyond computerised games, that I was concerned that he was over-relying on something destructive to cope with his own frustrations.' He paused. 'No, I wouldn't say that. I don't want to undermine what is helpful to him. I've got to sort out my attitude, but then, while I can offer him warm acceptance, I don't necessarily have to appear to agree with what he is doing.'

'Mhmm, but it sounds like you would feel a need to say something?'

'I would. I think it would be important.'

'For whom?'

'For ... hmm, well, I was going to say for Nick, but it's more for me, isn't it? I mean, I kind of want to hear myself saying something. I don't know, just seems like he's just being left to get on with his life at home and it feels like he's not getting much direction.'

'And you want to give him that direction?'

'No.' Simon realised immediately he had replied too quickly. 'Dammit, I guess I do. But I don't as well. Oh hell.'

'You do but you don't?' Sarida replied bluntly to maintain the edge that had arisen in the way Simon was talking.

'I-er, well, I want him to have direction, but I can't do that, I'm person-centred.'

Person-centered therapy was originally described in terms of being 'non-directive' therapy. This attitude of non-directivity remains an important feature of the approach even though it does not figure in the necessary and sufficient conditions of constructive personality change as described by Rogers (1957a).

'OK, let's get real on this. You, as a counsellor, don't want to be directive because that is at odds with the theoretical approach, but as a person you do want to be able to direct Nick, or at least contribute some influence on his choices?'

Simon listened to Sarida. He wanted to disagree with her, but he knew he agreed as well. Like different parts of himself were reacting to her words at the same time, generating conflict in himself.

'The truth is, I, as a man, want to have a positive influence on Nick. It's a father thing. I mean, I know how I was with my son, although he never really got that intensely into computer games; he was much more into sport and stuff like that at Nick's age. And my daughter, well, she's not interested in computers much, clothes and make-up, boys and CDs, that's where she's at, God help me.'

Sarida smiled. 'Having a tough time, huh?'

'Yeah.' He could also smile as well as he thought about her, how old she thought she was at the age of 15. Of course she was, almost old enough to be out to work now. Anyway, he got his thoughts back to Nick. 'I've got to watch myself, haven't I? I have an agenda here. I think it's the sense that Nick isn't getting much fathering and, well, yeah, there's a pull to get in there myself and make a difference. And I can't, not from that angle and motivation. I'm there as a

counsellor, someone for him to talk things through with. I wish his father could do that, but that's not what's happening. I'm kind of substituting, although I'm not because that's not my role. I have to listen, accept him as he is with all that he does, and help him come to terms with all that is happening in his life. I can at least model a way of relating between man and boy. I want that to be healthy and something that he can take with him into his future.'
'I hear how important that is, and yes, he will no doubt experience a contrast. I hope it won't confuse him.'
'I don't think so. I feel that he is intelligent enough to weigh things up, in spite of all that has happened. It's a difficult one, though, and I'll be mindful of it.'
'Yes, and I know I'm still feeling a certain wariness over your maybe responding to his need for fathering and finding it pushing you off your role.'
'It's a congruence issue as far as I'm concerned. It's my urge to father that is being tapped into here. I can see that and I need to carry that awareness into the sessions. I think that this is helping me to acknowledge it. It goes beyond the computer games. I just need to watch my boundaries but at the same time I need to try and avoid compromising my authenticity.'
Sarida nodded. 'Yes, the challenge though is to avoid authentically bringing your needs into the relationship.'
'Yeah. So many think congruence means "if I think it or I feel it, then I say it". But it isn't like that, is it?'
Sarida shook her head. 'No. Far from it.'
Simon went on to acknowledge his need to be open to his experiencing in the relationship and to maintain vigilance towards himself as to whether he might stray into a fathering reaction rather than counselling responses. He felt good about the discussion. He somehow felt clearer again. Once more, supervision had helped him disentangle stuff that he hadn't fully appreciated was even present for him. He wished this sort of collaborative working was more available to others in the caring professions whose work involved relationships with others.

So much difficulty could be avoided by some kind of reflective or collaborative review, enabling other professionals to be self-aware and avoid sliding into roles and responses that were the living out of their own needs, often to the detriment of the client who, when faced with incongruence in the therapist, tends to find their own incongruence rising, manifesting through greater confusion and anxiety.

Points for discussion

- Evaluate Simon's handling of Nick's initial silence and his being sick.
- Was Simon's response to Nick's disclosure regarding the attempted theft therapeutically helpful, and if so, why? What was happening from a person-centred theoretical perspective?

- How would you have handled Nick's 'wishing he was dead'? Was Simon right to let the session flow and come back to it later?
- If Nick had affirmed that he was suicidal with a plan in mind and an intent to act, what would you have done?
- Evaluate Sarida's style of supervision. Would you value it if you took your work to her?
- Write your own notes for counselling session 8.

CHAPTER 18

Counselling session 9: Nick finds satisfying experiences through music

'Still don't feel anyone cares at home.' Nick was looking down again and was feeling very low. Things were much better at school; he had made some more
friends the past week but he was being careful. These were other kids from the
music club, but they were more interested in music and that was something he
was feeling more and more drawn to. He hadn't really been into CDs and stuff
as much as other kids, preferring the games, but, well, yeah, he was liking some
of the stuff that they were listening to. He liked the power, the energy, and the
heavy nature of these bands that they were into. Kind of felt something stirring
inside himself when he listened to them.

The trouble was that as things got better at school he was feeling more pissed off
with how it was at home. And while the month ban on his games had really
become a struggle, the CDs he had been lent had compensated. Yeah, felt
good, got him away from feeling sorry for himself.

'Feels like your parents are not interested?'

Nick shook his head. 'No, they're still doing what they do and I kind of see them to
eat and, I don't know, just feels difficult. They don't seem to want to understand
me. Don't think they've forgiven me for, you know, trying to nick those cars.
Don't know what I can do to change them, don't think I can. Feels a waste
of time.'

'Mhmm, waste of time trying to change them. They just won't forgive you, yeah?'

Nick said nothing. He was just feeling so pissed off with it all. 'Just escape into my
music now.'

'That's become really important to you, the music.'

> Simon noted his curiosity as to what Nick was listening to, but he recognised
> this was his stuff and had no therapeutic significance, not at this stage
> anyway. Maybe later it might be of value to convey his interest, but at present
> the focus was on the importance of the music rather than the content.

Nick continued to be silent. He just felt fed up and didn't feel like saying anything. He just sat and stared at the carpet. A tune was going through his head; it had a really good bass and beat, and he liked that. He wanted to listen to stuff that had a bit of thump to it, an attitude, someone really giving the drums hell. Yeah, da-da-dada-dum, da-da-dada-dum, dadada dadada dada dum, dadada dadada dada dum. He hadn't realised his head was nodding to the imaginary beat in his head.

Simon watched Nick in his silence, the regular nodding motion, and guessed that he was preoccupied with something in his mind. He allowed Nick the space to be with what he was experiencing for a short while before commenting, 'Seems like you've got something in your head.' That sounded stupid, he thought, but it kind of said what he wanted to say.

'Yeah, just got a tune in my head, from this CD, this one track, it really builds up, you know, and it's got a really good beat, powerful, really makes me feel good.'

'Sounds great stuff. It really means a lot to you?'

'Yeah. Think I want to play something with power and rhythm, you know, can't be doing with the viola any more. Hasn't got enough guts, you know?'

'Mhmm, what you're listening to now has a kind of power, rhythm, guts that you can't get out of a viola. Different instrument, different experience, yeah?'

Nick nodded.

Simon was aware that he liked music that had a bit of power to it as well and he was still restraining his wanting to find out what album – do they still call them albums, he momentarily wondered – Nick was talking about.

Nick stayed silent a little longer, he had the tune back in his head again. Du-du-duu, dudu-dudu, du-du-duu, du-dudu. Yeah, felt good.

Simon had meanwhile decided to show interest in what Nick was interested in, but he wanted to do it in a way that wasn't invasive. He sensed the importance of music to Nick and he wanted to offer an appreciation of his interest and, per-haps, share in appreciation of the actual music. 'Guess I'm wondering what kind of music it is that's making such an impression on you.'

Simon is congruently expressing his curiosity. Is it appropriate to the coun-selling session? He feels it is as he is taking an interest in what is of interest to his client. He is offering an opportunity to communicate acceptance towards Nick and a developing part of his life that is important to him. Had the inter-vention been only motivated by curiosity then it would probably not have been appropriate.

'Hmm. Oh, a song from some band from the '70s, something about a fire. It's got a really great start, really powerful. I love it.'

'So, something about the power at the start. Really gives you something.'

'Yeah, it's just a guitar, and then it kind of builds on it and then, yeah, just makes me feel good, you know?'

Simon nodded. He could appreciate that kind of experience. He remembered the 1970s fondly, real music he always felt, but he knew everyone felt that about whichever era they were brought up in. He realised as well he was wondering what the song was. Would it be therapeutically helpful to try and find out? Well, it's about forming relationships with clients, and he knew from experience that often this meant a different approach when working with young people to the usual verbal exploration of thoughts, feelings, memories and events. Nick didn't have anyone really taking an interest in his hobbies. Maybe he could show that interest, and ... he heard Sarida in his head, and the discussion they had had about fathering. And he couldn't sit here thinking about it; he was there to focus on Nick. He decided to take further interest, take the risk of it coming across as fathering. Hell, Nick deserved someone showing interest in him, and it would give him a chance to explore the experience and maybe redefine himself within that experience.

'So, I'm sitting here wondering what the song is. I knew a few bands from that era.'

'The band's called Deep Purple, kind of different name. Ever heard of them?'

'Oh yes.' Simon smiled, too right he knew them. And he knew the song straight away, something of a Purple anthem, it had to be. 'So, you're talking about "Smoke on the Water"', huh?

'Yeah, that's it, yeah, how did you know?'

'It's the track that probably more than any other they are best known for. Yeah, it's powerful, and I can really appreciate now the impact it had on you.'

'Yeah, it feels so good, just, yeah, hard to describe, but it's the energy, you know, you can kind of get hold of it.' Nick was nodding. 'Yeah, it's great.'

Simon was still smiling. Funny old world, how things come around and back to you. 'Yeah, that song is about a fire. They were going to record something and someone burnt the building down.'

'Yeah, that's right. So, you ever seen them?'

'Yeah, a long time ago.' Simon felt that the focus was slipping into conversation but he decided to stay with it for a while longer. He had noticed Nick's face light up when he'd come up with the name of the song. That had felt a really important moment. He stayed with the topic. 'They're good, few line-up changes over the years, but always worth listening to.'

Sometimes the dialogue between client and counsellor can become conversational and remain therapeutic. It is dependent on the context, the nature of the relationship, the meaning for the client associated with the topic that is the focus of the conversation, and the motivation of the counsellor. Often as counselling moves towards an ending, greater conversation may emerge; however, it can have its place at other times. It can convey a sense of the personhood of the counsellor to the client, playing a part in equalising the power imbalance that arises between client and counsellor, although the person-centred approach seeks to minimise this.

'Can you recommend any other albums?' Nick was amazed that Simon knew about them. They must be good, he thought to himself.

'I think everyone has their own preferences. Some people prefer the early stuff, some the later. Some prefer studio albums, others prefer live performances.'

'Well, I'm gonna get some more. Just makes me feel alive. I can really get into it.'

'I guess we all need things to get into, and you've had the games, and now music's giving you a good feeling.'

'Yeah, funny that, it's all kind of come about a bit because of not being able to play the games. Probably wouldn't have borrowed the CD if I'd still been able to play them.' He paused. 'I'm kind of glad at what's happened, you know? Sort of feels good, somehow.'

'Something to feel good about, huh? It's so important to have that feeling.'

Nick sat back in silence, aware of feeling somehow better having just had the conversation he'd had. He didn't have the words to describe fully what he was experiencing, but he knew that he liked it. It felt like he was more alive, somehow, and he couldn't really explain it. But that was how it was. It just felt so good feeling that someone was taking an interest in him, in something that had become important to him. And it felt so good to share it, to talk about it. Talking as well to his two new friends, that felt really satisfying as well. Having something to talk about with them, yeah, he liked that. He hoped to get more into the music thing. He knew he'd still play the games, they were really important but, yeah, the music, that was really getting to him. And finding out that Simon knew that song, he smiled, amazing stuff.

Simon watched Nick, knowing that he was off in his own thoughts again. He must spend a lot of time in his own inner world, Simon thought, having spent so much time on his own. The part of him that communicates outside of himself is kind of evolving, emerging, and Simon felt a responsibility to help that process. And he also wanted to honour the internal dialogues that were probably taking place in Nick's head as well. It wasn't a case of one being better than the other: both were important features of Nick's nature.

A configuration is emerging within Nick in response to feeling listened to, and it has associated good feelings. This part of himself knows he is a person of worth, he has something to offer, something about himself that is of interest to others. His interest in music wasn't in order to gain friendship, or to gain a sense of positive worth from the reactions of others. The interest flourished and as a result he is discovering what it feels like to have a common interest in something. This contrasts with the part of his nature that believes himself to be not worth listening to, that is used to isolation and being verbally put down. It is a sensitive time for the client. The counsellor needs to be aware of this, to ensure that the configurational sense of self that is emerging is not distorted by 'conditions of worth' or unrealistic introjects.

The silence continued, broken by Nick saying, 'Not sure what else I want to talk about.'

'Nothing really pressing, nothing on your mind?'

He shook his head. Life felt better again. He didn't really feel he had any problems as he sat there. He had some good things going for him, although he also knew that there was the stuff at home in the background. But that felt less important somehow given the other changes in his life. And in a way, he didn't want to get into that anyway just now; he knew it would probably make him miserable and he didn't want that feeling. He wanted to feel like he was now, positive, with things to look forward to. The music had made a big difference, a big, big difference.

'Well, we've still got 20 minutes or so but, well, up to you what you want to do, Nick.'

'I'm kind of tempted to head off but then I kind of want to stay as well. I haven't got anything to really do, and it feels good being here talking about the kind of stuff we've talked about. But I don't know what to say, now. Feel kind of stuck.' He shrugged his shoulders.

'Stuck not knowing what to say.' Simon was aware as well of a sense of the contrast between how Nick was today and how he had been at the start, needing the sessions as a place of refuge. 'You're in a really different place to when I first saw you.'

It brought back to Nick how it had been. He nodded. 'I just needed somewhere to go. It was awful, and it really has changed out there.'

'Big change, out there and in you.'

'Yeah.'

They lapsed back into silence again. Nick didn't mind, somehow. His mind was wandering again across different things, but mainly the music, songs in his head, guitar riffs, drum beats.

Simon was aware of the temptation to suggest ending the session, but he was of the opinion that silence didn't mean time to end. Maybe Nick needed to be outwardly silent, although he sensed that in his head things were going on. Maybe being as he is but experiencing that in relationship with someone who's happy to allow it to be will also be of value. So he sat, with some eye contact on Nick, but also looking away from time to time as well, so as not to make it feel like he was under a kind of spotlight.

Nick was well into another song; in his head now, and had begun to tap the rhythm with his fingers. It was a fast song; it really had grabbed his attention. He loved the vocals on it as well, yeah, he'd got to a guitar solo in his head with a wonderful drum beat in the background. Yeah, he could really let himself go into it. Felt just so good.

Simon was smiling; he watched Nick tapping away. He's well away, he thought, and he looks different, calm, relaxed, like the worries have gone from his expression. He thought about saying this but chose to let Nick be with where he was and to say these things when Nick came out of the rhythm in his head.

A couple more minutes passed. Nick was at the end of the song. He was aware he was smiling and realised that he had really drifted off. He looked up, and Simon was looking at him with a big grin. He grinned back. 'Sorry. Well away there.'

'It was good to see. You looked engrossed and so relaxed.'

'I guess I was. Wasn't thinking about that, just got into another song.'

'Looked like a fast one, you were tapping out the rhythm.'

'Yeah, it's kind of growing on me. Called "Lazy", know it?'

'Uhu, so what's the album, *Machine Head, Made in Japan?*'

'*Made in Japan.*'

Simon nodded. 'Yeah, long tracks, time to really get into it. Quite an album to start with.'

'Yeah?'

'Yeah. And it really does make you feel good, doesn't it?'

'I can kind of forget everything. Bit like the games, but different as well.'

Simon wondered what the difference was. He conveyed that he had heard what Nick was saying, and he added a question which was present for him. 'Mhmm, forget everything. So it's similar but different, and I'm wondering what that difference is.'

Simon has not been really empathic here. He has picked up on what Nick has said but while his question has emerged out of his own experience, it has directed Nick away from the possibility of focusing on the similarities. There is perhaps a value judgement within Simon – unknown to him – that exploring differences may be more important than exploring similarities.

Nick thought about it. 'The games kind of take me away from stuff, but not really 'cos, you know, I've kind of got stuff in my head, particularly sometimes when I'm blasting the enemy. At least, that's how it has been. But the music, well, I'm just so focused on that and the rhythm and the sound and everything, I'm like not really thinking of anything. Like, yeah, it's just where I'm at and I just love it.'

'Great to have that and have that place in yourself, yeah, get away from it all and feel good. Gives you a break from stuff and a good feeling at the same time.'

Nick nodded.

Simon could see Nick getting more and more into this and in a way he could see it as a positive shift, and he could see that it might alienate him even more from his parents; he might find it left him more isolated in his head. But then, he's got a couple of new friends who are into the same thing, and so, yeah, that'll be a different experience, bit of social contact and, yeah, who knows what that'll lead to.

The session continued with another short period of silence before Nick commented that he felt ready to head off, but he wanted to keep coming to sessions. Simon said he was OK with that, and that maybe Nick could think about how he wanted to use the sessions in future, what more he wanted from them. Nick replied that he wasn't sure, but that it felt important and it left him feeling good, and he wanted more of that.

As Simon watched Nick go, he found himself thinking back to his own youth, the music he was into, and still listened to sometimes. It was later that evening when he dragged out his old copy of *Made in Japan* and played it – his wife was somewhat surprised and thought it was all a bit loud and noisy. But Simon wanted to reconnect with his own feelings from that time. Yeah, it still gave him a buzz, still felt the surge of energy and power. He ended up listening through the headphones to the two tracks that had been mentioned in the session, and it just took him away to another place in himself as well. He smiled to himself as he looked at the album sleeve – funny how clients can reconnect you to your own past. He knew he had to ensure his own feelings didn't dominate him in the sessions, but he also wanted to acknowledge to himself that, yeah, that music was still part of him after all these years.

That evening Nick was also listening to the CD he'd been loaned. Somehow the music felt even better now he had someone to talk to about it, who could remember the time when the album had first come out. That felt so good, so … he didn't know what it was, he couldn't put it into words, but it left him feeling more alive somehow. Yeah, he had something important in his life. Somehow the other hassles in his life seemed a little easier.

Points for discussion

- Was this a therapy session? What impact does it have on Nick?
- Would a therapist with a different interest in music have been more, or less, therapeutically helpful for Nick?
- Do you think that a more conversational style has particular value when working with young people?
- Do you feel the person-centred approach was being applied in this session and what is the basis for your conclusion?
- Do you feel optimistic for Nick?
- Looking back over the sessions with Simon so far, what were the critical points for the development of the therapeutic alliance?
- Write your own notes for this session.

Final reflections

Nick affirms his achievements and future goals

Nick was aware of the changes in himself that had happened since he had first come to counselling. He couldn't really explain them all, and he didn't really have the language to fully make sense of it or to communicate it, but he was aware of feeling somehow more freed up. He didn't have so much to worry about. The verbal bullying had stopped and it really felt great knowing he'd had a major part in stopping it. That felt quite powerful and he liked that. Yeah, he'd managed to silence them. The teachers, they'd taken him, it, seriously. It felt good to just walk along the corridor at school without always being tense, waiting for something to happen, listening out for footsteps. He still did sometimes, seemed to flip back into his old anxieties and worries. He had decided he wanted to talk to Simon about this in the next session. It wasn't a big deal, but he wanted to be sure that they would go. He didn't want them around at all.

He was also aware that he walked differently, had his head up more, felt more confident. That was at school, anyway. At home, well, things still weren't too easy. Still spent a lot of time in his room, but now listening more to music than to playing the games, though he still did the latter. But he didn't spend so much time at home now; he'd be round the houses of his two new friends, listening to music, talking about things. They all wanted to be able to play but weren't too sure about how to go about it. But they had all decided they'd try and get some instruments out of their parents for Christmas. Nick rather liked the idea of drumming but that seemed kind of a bit unlikely. But he liked rhythm and he was feeling drawn to bass guitar; he had found he could really pick out the bass rhythms in his head.

He didn't know how long the counselling would last; in fact, while he looked forward to it, somehow it didn't have the same importance to him. It was like he had other things going for him, but he didn't want to lose it just yet. He wanted to talk to Simon about different songs he was coming across, wanting to know if he knew them as well.

The stuff with his parents Nick wanted to do something about. He knew if he was going to get a guitar out of them he'd have to maybe be real good, so he was setting about that as well, trying to be a little more helpful round the house. He still got frustrated with their lack of real interest. He'd decided to ask his dad what kind of music he'd liked when he was younger, and see if there was any way of getting to know him better that way. He did want to have a better relationship with him. He wanted to be able to talk to him like he did with Simon.

Yeah, Nick thought to himself, life feels good. And he still had his lessons to think about as well. He didn't really like them much, and homework was a pain, but with his two friends they kind of were working on things together, talking it through and that felt great as well. All in all, things had changed for the better and ... he looked at the clock, shit, getting late. He turned off his CD player and went downstairs to find something to eat before going out to his friend's that afternoon. He was smiling ...

Simon reflects on what he feels has been achieved

Simon was aware that while, in one sense, he and Nick had not had many sessions, in his experience young people often did not want a counselling relationship that would go on for ages. They would come in with a problem looking for an immediate solution. In a very real sense, the problem that Nick had come to counselling about had been resolved. He was no longer experiencing the verbal bullying and abuse that had been very much part of his school experience. Simon was very pleased that it had all happened in the way that it had because it had clearly had a huge impact on the culture of the school and had actually generated what he sensed to be a real bonding among staff, and to a certain degree between staff and pupils.

He was also aware that Nick had made a big mistake with the attempted theft, and it seemed highly likely that he had learned from it. Yet it hadn't stopped him making new friends, and this expansion of his social world seemed to Simon extremely important. For Simon, the counselling relationship had moved on, and now it was about providing a therapeutic climate in which Nick could develop without the oppressive and distorting impact of the bullying. His self-esteem was lifting and, through the music, he was finding a way of feeling good about himself, and this was a resource other than the violent computer games that had previously been such a central feature of his life.

Nick was shifting away from the negative conditioning, from feeling useless, hopeless. He had recognised that he had power and was discovering what it was like to feel a sense of power within him. Yet the difficulties at home remained, although even there Nick seemed to have formulated a strategy to try and improve things. The very presence of this intention was reflective of the kind of self-belief that was beginning to emerge within him.

Simon wondered how his own way of being within the counselling sessions would have impacted on Nick. He had sought to listen, to engage with him, to accept what he had to say and how he was. He knew that he felt good about Nick; the positive regard he felt was genuine and, he thought, unconditional. He wasn't in any way experiencing any sense of only feeling good about Nick if he behaved a particular way. He didn't feel judgemental over the attempted theft. He had felt sad and sorry that it had happened, seeing the impact it had had on Nick. He appreciated that his parents had felt a need to take some action, but he hoped that the relationship with them would improve. He knew he wasn't party to the full family history, and he knew as well that he didn't need to be. He felt confident that so long as Nick could continue to experience a satisfying sense of self from his life, from the choices he was making, he would grow, mature and find ways of relating to his parents.

Of course, he knew as well that he was generally an optimist in life. Was he being unrealistic? He didn't think so. He couldn't be sure; the future was something to discover when it becomes the present, and not before. But he felt good about his work with Nick. He was still mindful of that fathering issue, and he knew he had to be careful, yet he didn't want to be so careful that he stopped being authentic and open. That wasn't the answer either. The truth is, he did want to make a difference in Nick's life and he was seeing that happen. He didn't want him to be a particular kind of person; he had no goal in mind for him, other than to have the opportunity to be free of the oppressive and damaging effect of the bullying and the overwhelming sense of powerlessness and low self-esteem that it could generate.

He was aware that those aspects of Nick's nature would remain with him, leaving him perhaps more sensitive to those experiences and feelings should they arise, or threaten to arise, in the future. But Nick now knew, from his own experience of himself, that he could feel, think and behave differently. He was realising that he had choices as to the life he wanted to lead – and that, thought Simon, is perhaps the most empowering experience that any young person can have, well, maybe the second most important. The most important was always going to be feeling consistently and unconditionally loved and lovable. That was always going to be the surest foundation for healthy psychological growth. As a person-centred counsellor, Simon was often aware that this was what he was offering the young people that he worked with – a place, a space, to feel cared for, to be offered authenticity and a chance to be understood. Relationship – right, healthy, wholesome relationship – Simon mused to himself. He felt himself smile inwardly: probably the most difficult thing to measure and quantify and yet the most powerful factor in the healing process.

Reflections from the author

Writing this book was a challenge from the start. Could I create characters that were believable? Would it convey something of the dynamic of the adult working with the young person, and the young person seeking help from an adult world? I hope that it has. I have felt deeply moved by the characters which, while fictional, nevertheless develop their own life as the writing proceeds. I have felt myself in all of the characters at different times in writing these two dialogues: the counsellors, their supervisors and, of course, the clients. And as I have been writing I have felt deeply moved as some of the sentences that they have spoken have emerged into my own thinking and taken shape on the page before me.

I know that I am not the person I was when I started out on this journey with these clients. It has required me to enter into an imaginary world, yet a world that for so many young people is all too real. As I reflect back now I realise that while I have been writing for counsellors and other professionals, hoping to offer them insight into a person-centred experience of working with young people, behind that is an important desire to write in a way that represents the needs of young people.

We live in difficult times, a society of great intensity, of fast everything, of materialistic emphasis. Young minds and hearts must sometimes feel like a battleground, caught in an advertising war and the constant pressure to perform at school through endless testing within the context of a society that says, 'You're good if you achieve'.

I am glad I am not a young person today with all the pressures placed upon them. I am pleased to have grown up in the late 1960s and early 1970s, which also had its problems and challenges. So I salute the young people today who are trying to find their way in the world, to discover values to live by that are not necessarily a blind following of the demands placed on them by society. My hope is that each young person has an opportunity to discover their own potential as adults in the making, and where they have experienced traumatic episodes, chaotic and uncertain upbringings, and a sense of feeling oppressed, whatever the cause, that they will have access to the kind of therapeutic environment and relationship that the person-centred approach offers. For me, as a person-centred counsellor, my motivation remains one of hoping that, in the encounter I have with my clients, a difference will be made, and a more whole, fulfilled and satisfied person will emerge as a result of that encounter.

References

Aspy DN (1965) *A study of three facilitative conditions and their relationship to the achievement of third grade students* (doctoral dissertation). University of Kentucky, KY. Unpublished.

Aspy DN (1967) Counseling and education. In: RR Cackhuff (ed.) *The Counselor's Contribution to Facilitative Processes*. Parkinson, Urbana, IL.

Aspy DN (1969) The effect of teacher-offered conditions of empathy, positive regard and congruence upon student achievement. *Florida Journal of Educational Research*. 11: 39–48.

Aspy DN and Hadlock W (1967) The effect of empathy, warmth, and genuineness on elementary students' reading achievement. Reviewed in: CB Truax and RR Carkhuff *Toward Effective Counseling and Psychotherapy*. Aldine, Chicago, IL.

Aspy DN and Roebuck FN (1970) *An investigation of the relationship between student levels of cognitive functioning and the teacher's classroom behavior* (manuscript). University of Florida, Gainsville, FL. Unpublished.

Bozarth J (1998) *Person-Centred Therapy: a revolutionary paradigm*. PCCS Books, Ross-on-Wye.

Bozarth J and Wilkins P (eds) (2001) *Rogers' Therapeutic Conditions: evolution, theory and practice*. Volume 3: *Congruence*. PCCS Books, Ross-on-Wye.

Everall RD and Paulson BL (2002) The therapeutic alliance: adolescent perspectives. *Counselling and Psychotherapy Research*. 2(2): 78–87.

Gaylin N (2001) *Family, Self and Psychotherapy: a person-centred perspective*. PCCS Books, Ross-on-Wye.

Haugh S and Merry T (eds) (2001) *Rogers' Therapeutic Conditions: evolution, theory and practice*. Volume 2: *Empathy*. PCCS Books, Ross-on-Wye.

Jenkins P (2002) Young peoples' rights to confidential therapy in the healthcare setting. *Healthcare Counselling and Psychotherapy Review*. 2: 11–14.

Kirschenbaum H and Henderson VL (eds) (1990) *The Carl Rogers Reader*. Constable, London.

Mearns D (1999) Person centred therapy with configurations of self. *Counselling*. 10: 125–30.

Mearns D and Thorne B (1988) *Person Centred Counselling in Action*. Sage, London.

Mearns D and Thorne B (1999) *Person Centred Counselling in Action* (2e). Sage, London.

Mearns D and Thorne B (2000) *Person Centered Therapy Today: new frontiers in theory and practice*. Sage, London.

Mental Health Foundation (1999) *Bright Futures: promoting children and young people's mental health*. Mental Health Foundation, London.

Merry T (2002) *Learning and Being in Person Centred Counselling* (2e). PCCS Books, Ross-on-Wye.

Moon SF (1966) Teaching the self. *Improving College and University Teaching.* **14**: 213–29.

Pierce R (1966) An investigation of grade-point average and therapeutic process variables (dissertation). University of Massachusetts, Amherst, MA. Unpublished. Reviewed in: RR Carkhuff and BG Berenson (1967) *Beyond Counseling and Therapy.* Holt, Rinehart and Winston, New York.

Rogers CR (1957a) The necessary and sufficient conditions of therapeutic personality change. *Journal of Consulting Psychology.* **21**: 95–103.

Rogers CR (1957b) Personal thoughts on teaching and learning. *Merrill-Palmer Quarterly.* **3**: 241–3. Reprinted in: H Kirschenbaum and VL Henderson (eds) (1990) *The Carl Rogers Reader.* Constable, London, pp. 301–4.

Rogers CR (1959) A theory of therapy, personality and interpersonal relationships as developed in the client-centred framework. In: S Koch (ed.), *Psychology: a study of a science.* Volume 3: *Formulations of the person and the social context.* McGraw-Hill, New York, pp. 219–35.

Rogers CR (1961) *On Becoming a Person.* Constable, London.

Rogers CR (1963) Learning to be free. In: SM Farber and RH Wilson (eds) *Conflict and Creativity: control of the mind, part 2.* McGraw-Hill, New York, pp. 268–88. Reprinted in: CR Rogers and B Stevens *et al.* (1967) *Person to Person: the problem of being human.* Real People Press, Moab, UT.

Rogers CR (1967) The interpersonal relationship in the facilitation of learning. In: R Leeper (ed.) *Humanizing Education.* NEA, Washington, DC, pp. 1–18. Reprinted in: H Kirschenbaum and VL Henderson (eds) (1990) *The Carl Rogers Reader.* Constable, London, pp. 304–22.

Rogers CR (1969) *Freedom to Learn: a view of what education might become.* Charles E Merrill Publishing Co, Columbus, OH.

Rogers CR (1977) The politics of education. *Journal of Humanistic Education.* **1**: 6–22. Reprinted in: H Kirschenbaum and VL Henderson (eds) (1990) *The Carl Rogers Reader.* Constable, London, pp. 323–34.

Rogers CR (1980) *A Way of Being.* Houghton Mifflin, Boston, MA.

Rogers CR (1986) A client-centered/person-centered approach to therapy. In: I Kutash and A Wolfe (eds) *Psychotherapists' Casebook.* Jossey Bass, San Francisco, CA. pp. 197–208.

Schmuck R (1966) Some aspects of classroom social climate. *Psychology in the School.* **3**: 59–65.

Warner M (2002) Psychological contact, meaningful process and human nature. In: G Wyatt and P Sanders (eds) *Rogers' Therapeutic Conditions: evolution, theory and practice.* Volume 4: *Contact and Perception.* PCCS Books, Ross-on-Wye, pp. 76–96.

Wilkins P (2003) *Person Centred Therapy in Focus.* Sage, London.

Wyatt G (ed.) (2001) *Rogers' Therapeutic Conditions: evolution, theory and practice.* Volume 1: *Congruence.* PCCS Books, Ross-on-Wye.

Wyatt G and Sanders P (eds) (2002) *Rogers' Therapeutic Conditions: evolution, theory and practice.* Volume 4: *Contact and Perception.* PCCS Books, Ross-on-Wye.

Further reading

- Association of Nurses in Substance Abuse (1997) *Working with Children and Young People: Substance Use. Guidance on Good Clinical Practice for Nurses, Midwives and Health Visitors.* ANSA, London.

- Bryant-Jefferies R (2001) *Counselling the Person Beyond the Alcohol Problem.* Jessica Kingsley Publishers, London.

- Bryant-Jefferies R (2002) *Counselling a Recovering Drug User: a person-centred dialogue.* Radcliffe Medical Press, Oxford.

- DrugScope and Department of Health (2002) *Taking Care with Drugs: responding to substance use among looked after children.* DrugScope, London.

- DrugScope (2003) *First Steps in Identifying Young People's Substance Related Needs.* Drug Strategy Directorate, London.

- Standing Conference on Drug Abuse and the Children's Legal Centre (1999) *Young People and Drugs: policy guidance for drug interventions.* SCODA, London.

- Standing Conference on Drug Abuse (2000) *Assessing Young People's Drug Taking: guidance for drug services.* SCODA, London.

Useful contact

Talk to Frank
A national, free and confidential drugs information and advice service for young people, 24 hours a day – Talk to Frank.
Tel: 0800 77 66 00
Website: www.talktofrank.com
Email: frank@talktofrank.com
If you are deaf, textphone FRANK on 0800 917 8765.

Index